Let's talk about

SEX

MORE THAN
600 QUOTES
ON THE
WORLD'S OLDEST
OBSESSION

by

Felicia Zopol

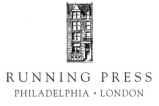

RUNNING PRESS
PHILADELPHIA · LONDON

9   8   7   6   5   4   3   2   1
Digit on the right indicates the number of this printing

Library of Congress Cataloging-in-Publication Number 2002108935

ISBN 0-7624-1453-7
Cover Photograph © Digital Stock, altered by Bill Jones
Interior Illustrations by Mielo So
Cover and interior design by Rosemary Tottoroto
Edited by Greg Jones
Typography: Garamond and Gill Sans

This book may be ordered by mail from the publisher.
Please include $2.50 for postage and handling.
But try your bookstore first!

Running Press Book Publishers
125 South Twenty-second Street
Philadelphia, Pennsylvania 19103-4399

Visit us on the web!
www.runningpress.com

CONTENTS

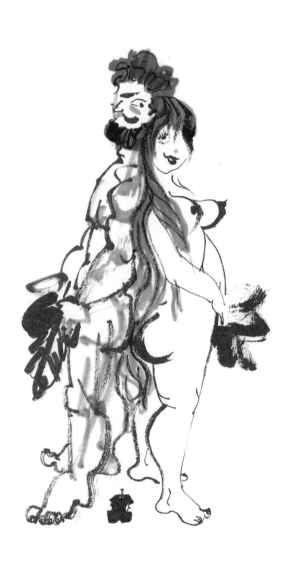

INTRODUCTION

Sex is timeless.

Fads come and go. Fashions evolve quickly and surely, and just as surely they disappear. Today's superstars, big hits, and news sensations inevitably fade into punch lines for tomorrow's nightclub comedians. (Let's talk about Monica Lewinsky and Heidi Fleiss? I don't think so!)

But sex has remained atop the charts of mankind's obsessions— Number One with a bullet bra—for over 10,000 years. Indeed, humanity's fascination with sex remains as strong as when Adam and Eve first took a long, hard look at one another and dared to speak the naked truth.

A lot has been said since on the subject of sex. Much of it profound, hilarious, titillating, and revealing. Here is a collection of history's choicest quotations on sex and its many themes, varieties, and implications.

The sources range as wide and wild as the topics, with entries from comedians, philosophers, musicians, sex surveys, medieval theologians and more. Hell, there are even quotes inside from Monica Lewinsky and Heidi Fleiss!

And why not? All sorts of people from all walks of life have their own perspective on the subject, as well as an insatiable curiosity to read what others have to say about the world's oldest obsession.

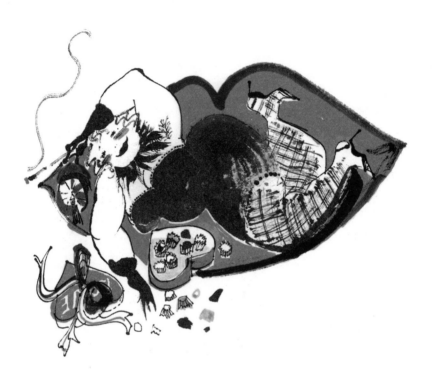

SEDUCTION AND TEMPTATION

Even most sexual gluttons and Kama Sutra
enthusiasts spend a lot more time looking
over the menu than enjoying the actual
feast of sexual experience. Some philosophers
and psychologists even claim that seduction
and the quest to satisfy sexual temptation
takes up most of our lives. While that
probably depends on the individual, there
has undoubtedly been a great deal said by a
great many individuals on how to attract a lover.
And what to do once you get one...

When I find a woman attractive, I have nothing at all to say. I simply watch her smile.

ANTOINE DE SAINT-EXUPERY (1900–1944)
French aviator, writer

I can resist everything but temptation.

OSCAR WILDE (1854–1900)
Irish Playwright

Lead me not into temptation. I can find the way myself.

RITA MAE BROWN (B. 1944)
American writer

One woman I was dating said, "Come on over, there's nobody home." I went over—nobody was home.

RODNEY DANGERFIELD (B. 1922)
American comedian

When you want your boyfriend to play with you, wear a full-length black nightgown with buttons all over it. Sure it's uncomfortable. But it makes you look just like his remote control.

DIANA JORDAN AND PAUL SEABURN
American humorists

He gave her a look you could have poured on a waffle.

RING LARDNER (1885–1933)
American writer, humorist

Glances are the heavy artillery of the flirt: everything can be conveyed in a look, yet that look can always be denied, for it cannot be quoted word for word.

STENDHAL (1783–1842)
French writer

Look at her. All over. Linger anywhere you like. When she notices (and she will if you're really looking), hold her eyes with yours. Hold them close. This is the essence of cruising, the experience that all the virtual reality and phone sex in the world will never replace. It is also the moment of truth. You'll know then and there whether she wants you or not.

SUSIE BRIGHT (B. 1958)
American writer, editor

You know that look women get when they want sex? Me neither.

DREW CAREY (B. 1958)
American comedian, actor

I have such poor vision I can date anybody.

GARY SHANDLING (B. 1949)
American comedian, actor

She gave me a smile I could feel in my hip pocket.

RAYMOND CHANDLER (1888–1959)
American writer

How well a soft and libertine voice will erect your member, it is as good as fingers.

JUVENAL (C. 60–140)
Roman writer

A man falls in love through his eyes, a woman through her ears.

WOODROW WYATT (B. 1918)
British journalist

To speak of love is to make love.

HONORE DE BALZAC (1799–1850)
French novelist

Ask, and ask sexy. Say "can I kiss you?" or "I'm feeling like we oughta take off all our clothes, grind our genitals together for twenty or so minutes, then hop back in the shower for a rinse and some cunnilingus, then jump back in bed, eat some Ben & Jerry's Cherry Garcia and then maybe have another go at it. How are you feeling?"

DAN SAVAGE
American sex-advice columnist

How many times have you started dating someone because you were too lazy to commit suicide?

JUDY TENUTA
American comedian

9

ALL REALLY GREAT LOVERS ARE ARTICULATE, AND VERBAL SEDUCTION IS THE SUREST ROAD TO ACTUAL SEDUCTION.

MARYA MANNES (1904–1990)
American journalist

You don't have to have a language in common with someone for a sexual rapport. But it helps if the language you don't understand is Italian.

MADONNA (B. 1958)
American pop star

That woman speaks eighteen languages and can't say, "No" in any of them.

DOROTHY PARKER (1893–1967)
American writer, humorist

The golden rule is to keep it simple. Don't try to over-explain who you are and how you're feeling. It's a frozen moment in amber. It's a small piece of your soul. Give her a taste—the little pink spoon, not the whole sundae.

JON FAVREAU (B. 1966)
American actor, screenwriter

VINCE VAUGHN (B. 1970)
American actor

I love the lines men use to get us into bed. "Please, I'll only put it in for a minute." What am I, a microwave?

BEVERLY MICKINS
American comedian

Sex is not the answer. Sex is the question. "Yes" is the answer.

ANONYMOUS

There's nothing worse than the girl who is considered charmless, except the man who is considered harmless.

EVAN ESAR (1899–1995)
American writer

You know what charm is: a way of getting the answer "yes" without having asked any clear question.

ALBERT CAMUS (1913–1960)
French writer, philosopher

I conclude that musical notes and rhythms were first acquired by the male and female progenitors of mankind for the sake of charming the opposite sex.

CHARLES DARWIN (1809–1882)
English naturalist

In Mexico, a bachelor is a man who can't play the guitar.

LILLIAN DAY (20TH CENTURY)
American playwright

Rock is really about dick and testosterone. I go see a band. I want to fuck the guy. That's the way it is. It's always been that way.

COURTNEY LOVE (B. 1964)
American musician, actress

Dancing is wonderful training for girls, it's the first way you learn to guess what a man is going to do before he does it.

CHRISTOPHER MORLEY (1890–1957)
American writer, editor

Guaranteed Effective Pickup Lines: Uh, like let's drop the B.S. and like, you know, do it.

MIKE JUDGE, CHRIS MARCIL,
AND SAM JOHNSON
From Beavis and Butthead's This Book Sucks!

Power is the ultimate aphrodisiac.

HENRY KISSINGER (B. 1923)
German-born American secretary of state

I like watching a man boss everybody around. It's so sexy.

ROBIN TUNNEY (B. 1972)
American actress

I know there are nights when I have power, when I put on something and walk in somewhere and if there is a man who doesn't look at me, it's because he's gay.

KATHLEEN TURNER (B. 1954)
American actress

"Where should one use perfume?" a young woman asked. "Wherever one wants to be kissed," I said.

COCO CHANEL (1883–1971)
French fashion designer

Oysters are supposed to enhance your sexual performance, but they don't work for me. Maybe I put them on too soon.

GARY SHANDLING (B. 1949)
American comedian, actor

I HAVE OBSERVED, ON BOARD A STEAMER,

HOW MEN AND WOMEN EASILY GIVE WAY

TO THEIR INSTINCT FOR FLIRTATION,

BECAUSE WATER HAS THE POWER OF WASHING

AWAY OUR SENSE OF RESPONSIBILITY,

AND THOSE WHO ON LAND RESEMBLE

THE OAK IN THEIR FIRMNESS BEHAVE

LIKE FLOATING SEAWEED WHEN ON THE SEA.

RABINDRANATH TAGORE (1861–1941)
Bengali poet, philosopher

Why are women wearing perfumes that smell like flowers? Men don't like flowers. I've been wearing a great new scent guaranteed to attract men. It's called New Car Interior.

RITA RUDNER (B. 1955)
American Comedian

There are a number of mechanical devices which increase sexual arousal, particularly in women. Chief among these is the Mercedes-Benz 380SL convertible.

P.J. O'ROURKE (B. 1947)
American writer and editor

You can seduce a man without taking anything off, without even touching him.

RAE DAWN CHONG (B. 1962)
American actress

I find it very difficult to draw a line between what's sex and what isn't. It can be very, very sexy to drive a car, and completely unsexy to flirt with someone at a bar.

BJORK GUDMUNDSDOTTIR (B. 1965)
Icelandic musician

Why does a man take it for granted that a girl who flirts with him wants him to kiss her—when, nine times out of ten, she only wants him to [want] to kiss her.

HELEN ROWLAND (1875–1950)
American journalist

Good sex begins when your clothes are still on.

WILLIAM MASTERS (1915–2001)
American sex researcher, writer

VIRGINIA JOHNSON (B. 1925)
American sex researcher, writer

My advice to those who think they have to take off their clothes to be a star is once you're boned, what's left to create the illusion? Let 'em wonder.

MAE WEST (1893–1980)
American actress

Sex appeal is 50 percent what you've got and 50 percent what people think you've got.

SOPHIA LOREN (B. 1934)
Italian actress

The longer they wait, the better they like it.

MARLENE DIETRICH (1901–1992)
German actress

In the art of love it is more important to know when than how.

EVAN ESAR (1899–1995)
American writer

I set out to seduce [her]. I tried the only way I could think of: by loitering.

JOSEPH HELLER (1923–1999)
American writer

The longest absence is less perilous to love than the terrible trials of incessant proximity.

OUIDA (1839–1908)
French writer

An absence, the declining of an invitation to dinner, an unintentional, unconscious harshness are of more service than all the cosmetics and fine clothes in the world.

MARCEL PROUST (1871–1922)
French writer

It is easier to keep half a dozen lovers guessing than to keep one lover after he has stopped guessing.

HELEN ROWLAND (1875–1950)
American journalist

*What else do women
want in life but to be as
attractive as possible to men?
Do not all their trimmings and
cosmetics have this end in view,
and all their baths, fittings,
creams, scents, as well—
and all those arts of making up,
painting and fashioning the
face, eyes and skin.
And by what other sponsor
are they better recommended
to men than by folly?*

ERASMUS (C. 1469–1536)
Dutch priest, humanist and scholar

Sometimes they wore
Kiss makeup, sometimes
I did. Many times beauties
have wanted to sleep
with the beast.

GENE SIMMONS (B. 1949)
American rock star

To win a date with me,
one guy lay in a bed of
cockroaches for four hours.
I think he deserved it.

SOFIA VERGARA (B. 1972)
Colombian model, actress

I have the knack of
easing scruples.

MOLIÈRE (1622–1672)
French playwright

Most virtue is demand
for greater seduction.

NATALIE CLIFFORD BARNEY
(1878–1972)
American writer

In a blush, love finds
a barrier.

VIRGIL (70–19 [SC]B.C.)
Roman poet

**Whoever blushes is already guilty, true innocence
is ashamed of nothing.**

JEAN JACQUES ROSSEAU (1712–1778)
French writer, philosopher

It is assumed that the
woman must wait, motion-
less, until she is wooed.
That is how the spider waits
for the fly.

GEORGE BERNARD SHAW (1856–1950)
Irish playwright

To seduce a woman
famous for strict morals,
religious fervor and the
happiness of her marriage:
what could possibly be
more prestigious?

CHRISTOPHER HAMPTON (B. 1946)
British playwright

He wondered why sexual
shyness, which excites the
desire of dissolute women,
arouses the contempt of
decent ones.

COLETTE (B. 1934)
French writer

The bashful hog eats
no pears.

ITALIAN PROVERB

There are several good protections against temptations, but the surest is cowardice.

MARK TWAIN (1835–1910)
American writer, lecturer and humorist

"Come to the edge," he said.
They said, "We are afraid."
"Come to the edge," he said.
They came. He pushed
them…and they flew.

APOLLINAIRE (1880–1918)
French writer

Temptation discovers
what we are.

THOMAS A KEMPIS (1379-80–1471)
German monk, writer

Anybody who knows
Dan Quayle knows
that he would rather
play golf than have
sex any day.

MARILYN QUAYLE (B. 1949)
*American Second Lady, responding to
charges that her husband had an affair
while on a golf vacation*

It is a stroke of good
fortune to find one
who is worth seducing…
Most people rush ahead,
become engaged or do
other stupid things. And in
a turn of the hand, everything is over, and they know
neither what they have won,
nor what they have lost.

SORËN KIERKEGAARD (1813–1855)
Danish philosopher

The awful daring of
a moment's surrender,
which an age of prudence
can never retract.
By this and only this
we have existed.

T.S. ELIOT (1888–1965)
British poet From "The Wasteland"

We have been raised
to fear the "yes" within
ourselves, our deepest
cravings. For the
demands of our released
expectations lead us
inevitably into actions
which will help bring our
lives into accordance
with our needs, our
knowledge, our desires.

AUDRE LORDE (1934–1992)
American poet

16

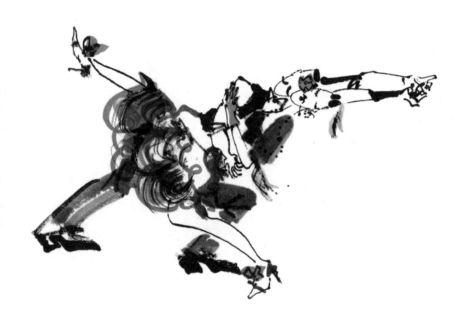

THE ACT

Coition. The Nasty. Cunnilingus. Head.

The most common terms used to describe

sex acts tend to be clumsy and academic,

or short and none-too-sweet. It's as if you

had to choose between going to bed with a

lab-bound egghead or a street-corner thug.

Fortunately, poets, philosophers, and all manner

of regular folk have also occasionally weighed

in on the subject, revealing that the language

and thematic possibilities of sexual activity

are as rich and deep as the feelings they inspire.

Arousal is a miracle... an unsolicited endorsement, a standing ovation, a spontaneous demonstration.

PLAYBOY, DECEMBER 1981

Sex is not something we do, it is something we are.

MARY CALDERONE (1904–1998)
American physician, sex educator, writer

I'm suggesting we call sex something else, and it should include everything from kissing to sitting close together.

SHERE HITE (B. 1942)
American sex writer, researcher

Her kisses left something to be desired— the rest of her.

ANONYMOUS

He was the kind of guy who could kiss you behind your ear and make you feel like you'd just had kinky sex.

JULIA ALVAREZ (B. 1950)
American writer

He moved his lips about her ears and neck as though in thirsting search for an erogenous zone. A waste of time, he knew from experience. Erogenous zones are either everywhere or nowhere.

JOSEPH HELLER (1923–1999)
American writer

I am not so easily aroused. For me it takes quite a long time until the first kiss.

JENNIFER LOPEZ (B. 1970)
American actress, singer

He was every other inch a gentleman.

REBECCA WEST (1892–1983)
British writer, critic

A gentleman doesn't pounce, he glides.

QUENTIN CRISP (1908–1999)
British writer, actor

Some men know that a light touch of the tongue, running from a woman's toes to her ears, lingering in the softest way possible in various places in between, given often and sincerely enough, would add immeasurably to world peace.

MARIANNE WILLIAMSON (B. 1952)
American writer, lecturer

Love is blind; that is why it always proceeds by the sense of touch.

FRENCH PROVERB

Sexual relationships are often like an hourglass; one single point of contact.

BERNARD BERENSON (1865–1959)
American writer, critic

Anyone who calls it "sexual intercourse" can't possibly be interested in doing it. You might as well announce that you're ready for lunch by proclaiming, "I'd like to do some masticating and enzyme secreting."

ALLAN SHERMAN (1924–1973)
American television writer, comedian and musician

I sing the body eclectic. I marvel at the poignancy of a mercy fuck on the living-room couch. I amaze at the doggy-style extravaganza in the bathroom of a 757. I blush at the latest Kama Sutra position, the Begging Yoni. Sex is a circus with a cute ringleader, a virtual Chinese restaurant of choices....

CYNTHIA HEIMEL
American writer, humorist

To lovers, touch is metamorphosis. All the parts of their bodies seem to change, and seem to become something different and better.

JOHN CHEEVER (1912–1982)
American writer

Now that I think of it,
the sweetest outdoor tryst
I ever had...was the time
a very nice girl gave me
body surfing lessons.
Every time a wave came up to us
that we couldn't catch, and I'd get scared,
she'd tell me to hold her hands,
kiss her and duck/dive down
under until it passed over us.
I didn't have a human being orgasm,
but I think I had a mermaid one,
and that's the sort of thing you
would like to look forward to
when you leave the comfort
and safety of your
bedroom behind.

SUSIE BRIGHT (B.1958)
American writer, editor

"Sex" is as important as eating or drinking and we ought to allow the one appetite to be satisfied with as little restraint or false modesty as the other.

MARQUIS DE SADE (1740–1814)
French author.

I need more sex, okay? Before I die, I wanna taste everyone in the world.

ANGELINA JOLIE (B. 1975)
American actress

The ability to make love frivolously is the chief characteristic which distinguishes human beings from the beasts.

HEYWOOD BROUN (1888–1939)
American journalist

They made love as though they were an endangered species.

PETER DE VRIES (B. 1910)
American writer

In love, as in gluttony, pleasure is a matter of the utmost precision.

ITALO CALVINO (1923–1985)
Cuban-Italian writer

I feel like a million tonight—just one at a time.

MAE WEST (1893–1980)
American actress

I would love to have sex all the time, even in the swimming pool. I don't care if it's the deep end or the shallow. I can work anyplace.

JULIO IGLESIAS (B.1943)
Spanish singer

Sex is part of nature. I go along with nature.

MARILYN MONROE (1926–1962)
American actress

Sex, on the whole, was meant to be short, nasty and brutish. If what you want is cuddling, you should buy a puppy.

JULIE BURCHILL (B. 1960)
British writer

It was lovemaking, Doctor, even though it was nasty. Maybe especially because it was nasty. Love is smutty business, you know.

TOM ROBBINS (B. 1936)
American writer

I WAS BEYOND SIMPLE DESIRE,
BORNE AWAY RATHER BY A NEAR SWOON
OF LUST. COULDN'T SHE KNOW WHAT SHE
DID TO ME WITH THIS CONCUBINE
SPEECH, WITH THESE FOUL,
PRICELESS WORDS WHICH ASSAIL LIKE
SHARP SPEARS THE BASTION OF MY OWN
CHRISTIAN GENTILITY WITH ITS ARCHING
REPRESSIONS AND RESTRAINTS.

WILLIAM STYRON (B. 1925)
American writer

Whatever else can be said about sex, it cannot be called a dignified performance.

HELEN LAWRENSON (1907–1982)
American writer, editor

Sex is making a fool of yourself…. That is why sex is so intimate. Making mistakes is one of the most revealing and intimate moments of sexual communication.

JERRY RUBIN (1938–1994)
American journalist, therapist

…on the level of simple sensation and mood, making love surely resembles having an epileptic fit at least as much as, if not more than, it does eating a meal or conversing with someone.

SUSAN SONTAG (B. 1933)
American writer

Sex is a conversation carried out by another means.

PETER USTINOV (B. 1921)
British writer, actor

I have made love to ten thousand woman since I was thirteen-and-a-half. It wasn't in any way a vice. I have no sexual vices. But I needed to communicate.

GEORGE SIMENON (1903–1989)
Belgian writer

The language of sex is yet to be invented. The language of the senses is yet to be explored.

ANAIS NIN (1903–1977)
French writer

What do atheists scream when they come?

BILL HICKS (1961–1994)
American comedian

The most romantic thing a woman ever said to me in bed was, "Are you sure you're not a cop?"

LARRY BROWN
American comedian

A woman should be obscene, and not heard.

GROUCHO MARX (1895–1977)
American entertainer

I don't say anything during sex. I've been told not to. Told during sex in fact.

CHEVY CHASE (B. 1943)
American actor, comedian

Oral sex is currently very trendy. It is even preferred to the regular kind. It is preferred because it's the only way most of us can get our sex partners to shut up.

P.J. O'ROURKE (B. 1947)
American writer, editor

I swear people don't want sex so much as they want somebody who'll listen to 'em… the first thing you learn after fellatio is how to listen.

JANE WAGNER (B. 1935)
American writer, actress and director

To see, taste, touch, hear and smell the essence of a woman is to become a successful explorer, a modern Jacques Cousteau, a teacher and an A-plus student, all at the same time.

DYLAN EDWARDS
American writer

Some men love oral sex…. If you find a man like this, treat him well. Feed him caviar and don't let your girlfriends catch a glimpse of him.

CYNTHIA HEIMEL
American writer, humorist

Made a hell of a discovery the other night. Eyelashes on the clit…can blink her off in no time.

DAN JENKINS (B.1929)
American novelist and journalist

…It's so easy where it is and men never seem to be able to find it. You're like, 'It's right there!' When they do find it, you wish that they hadn't because they're really rough…they're pushing it like it's an elevator button.

JENNIFER TILLY (B. 1958)
Canadian-born American actress

Is sex dirty?
Only if it's done right.

WOODY ALLEN (B. 1935)
American filmmaker, actor and writer

For male and female alike, the bodies of the other sex are messages signaling what we must do—they are glowing signifiers of our own necessities.

JOHN UPDIKE (B. 1932)
American author, critic

It's really time for us to grow up and discover our vaginas.

LORETTA SWIT (B. 1937)
American actress

Really, that little dealybob is too far away from the hole. It should be built right in.

LORETTA LYNN (B. 1935)
American singer-songwriter

It was never dirty to me. After all, God gave us the equipment and the opportunity. There's that old saying, "If God had meant us to fly, he'd have given us wings." Well, look what he did give us.

DOLLY PARTON (B. 1946)
American singer-songwriter

God, how I envied girls....
Whatever it was on them, it didn't
dangle between their legs like an
elephant trunk. No wonder boys talked
about nothing but sex.
That thing was always there.
Every time I went to the john,
there it was, twitching around like
a little worm on a fishing hook.
When we took baths, it floated
around in the water like a lazy fish,
and God forbid we should touch it.
It sprang to life like lightning
leaping from a cloud.

JULIUS LESTER (B. 1939)
American writer

Contrary to Freud's theory, we do not envy the penis. The reasons are obvious. First, we would not know how to sit comfortably with one; second, we do not want something veiny falling out of our shorts; and third, a penis looks terrible in a tight dress.

ANKA RADAKOVITCH
American sex columnist

I have a little bit of penis envy. Yeah they're ridiculous, but they're cool.

K.D. LANG (B. 1962)
Canadian-born American singer

If the world were a logical place, men would ride side saddle.

RITA MAE BROWN (B. 1944)
American writer

War is menstrual envy.

RUTH MARCOZZI (B. 1951)
American advice columnist

Sexual passion is the cause of war and the end of peace, the basis of what is serious… and consequently the concentration of all desire.

ARTHUR SCHOPENHAUER
(1788–1860)
German philosopher

Sex is only interesting when it releases passion. The more extreme and the more expressed that passion is, the more unbearable does life seem without it. It reminds us that if passion dies or is denied, we are partly dead and that soon, come what may, we will be wholly so.

JOHN BOORMAN (B. 1933)
British filmmaker

Eroticism is assenting to life, even to the point of death.

GEORGE BATAILLE (1897–1962)
French writer

It would have been good to die at any moment then, for love and death had somewhere joined hands.

LAWRENCE DURRELL (1912–1990)
British writer

Bury me, bury me
Deeper, ever so deeper.
ALFRED LORD TENNYSON (1809–1892)
British poet

After we made love he took a piece of chalk and made an outline of my body.

JOAN RIVERS (B. 1937)
American comedian

There will be sex after death—we just won't be able to feel it.
LILY TOMLIN (B. 1939)
American comedian

I may not be a great actress but I've become the greatest at screen orgasms—ten seconds' heavy breathing, roll your head from side to side, simulate a slight asthma attack and die a little.
CANDACE BERGEN (B. 1946)
American actress

How alike are the groans of love to those of the dying.
MALCOLM LOWRY (1909–1957)
British writer

It may be discovered someday that an orgasm actually lasts for hours and only seems like a few seconds.
DOLLY PARTON (B. 1946)
American singer-songwriter

I once made love for an hour and fifteen minutes. But it was the night the clocks were set ahead.
GARY SHANDLING (B. 1949)
American comedian, writer, actor

The position is ridiculous, the pleasure momentary, the expense damnable.
LORD CHESTERFIELD (1694–1773)
British writer

Electric flesh-arrows...traversing the body. A rainbow of color strikes the eyelids. A foam of music falls over the ears. It is the gong of the orgasm.
ANAIS NIN (1903–1977)
French writer

THE ACT

All this fuss about sleeping together. For physical pleasure I'd sooner go to my dentist any day.

EVELYN WAUGH (1903–1966)
British writer

I'm a terrible lover. I've actually given a woman an anti-climax.

SCOTT ROEBEN (B. 1965)
American writer

If it happens that you do want peanut butter in bed while you're having sex and your partner doesn't, in the long run the thing to do may be to find another partner.

DR. RUTH WESTHEIMER (B. 1928)
German-born American sex therapist and author

I once had a rose named after me and I was very flattered. But I was not pleased to read the description in the catalog: no good in a bed, but fine up against a wall.

ELEANOR ROOSEVELT (1884–1962)
American diplomat, first lady

People have come up with kinky sex because it's memorable…. When you do something kinky, it's like, yes, the mango sex. We'll always remember the mango sex. Try it, but try it with a sheet you can throw away, because there's nothing stickier than mango sex. It wasn't even that good, but we remember it. And that's the key—the remembering.

BETH LAPIDES
American comedian

I'd like to meet the man who invented sex and see what he's working on now.

ANONYMOUS

There's nothing better than good sex. But bad sex? A peanut butter and jelly sandwich is better than bad sex.

BILLY JOEL (B. 1949)
American musician

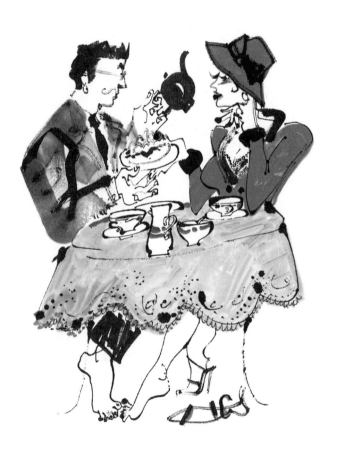

MANNERS AND MORALITY

Sex serves as humanity's ultimate ethical minefield.
Thousands of taboos have been nominated for normalcy
over the ages and across the globe. Yet almost none
of them have gained universal acceptance, or even
consistent enforcement within their own societies.
Indeed, what some cultures and individuals consider
sin, serves as recreation and added spice to others.
Of course, this vast gray area hasn't stopped everyone
from ancient prophets to modern-day advice
columnists from trying to stake out the blacks and
whites, dos and don'ts, rights and wrongs, and moral
absolutes of sexual relationships. Guess we have to
keep looking, and pushing the envelope in the meantime.

Faithfulness is to the emotional life what consistency is to the life of the intellect— simply a confession of failure.

OSCAR WILDE (1854–1900)
Irish Playwright

I keep making up these sex rules for myself, and then I break them right away.

J. D. SALINGER (B. 1919)
American writer

There are only two guidelines for good sex, "Don't do anything you don't really enjoy," and "Find out your partner's needs and don't balk at them if you can help it."

DR. ALEX COMFORT (1920–2000)
British writer, sexologist

It's okay to laugh in the bedroom so long as you don't point.

WILL DURST
American satirist

Southerners will forgive anybody anything if they have good manners. Once a particularly charming Congressman who had been a guest at a church dinner my mother had attended was caught sometime later rather, well, flagrantly, as the French would say, in a motel room wearing a dog collar and his wife's lace bra and panties. Mother's response when asked if she would vote for him again? "Why, of course. After all, everybody's got their little quirks. Besides he has lovely table manners."

FANNIE FLAGG (B. 1944)
American actress, writer

34

You sleep with a guy
once and before you
know it he wants to take
you to dinner.

MYERS YORI
American writer

It would be rude to
get your sexual satisfaction
by tying someone
to the bed and then
leaving him or her there
and going out with
someone more
attractive.

P.J. O'ROURKE (B. 1947)
American writer, editor

It is an irony, appreciated
only by the French,
that good manners are
the basis of very good
sex. In bed, the two most
erotic words in any
language are "thank you"
and "please."

HUBERT DOWNS

Responding to suggestion
that he take a wife:
With all my heart.
Whose wife shall it be?

JOHN HORNE TOOKE (1736–1812)
British politician

**I consider
promiscuity immoral.
Not because sex
is evil, but because
sex is too good and
important.**

AYN RAND (1905–1982)
Russian-American writer

When choosing
between two evils,
I always take the one
I haven't tried before.

MAE WEST (1893–1980)
American actress

The resistance of a
woman is not always a
proof of her virtue,
but more frequently
of her experience.

NINON DE LENCLOS (C. 1620–1705)
French writer

**I say I don't sleep with married men,
but what I mean is that I don't sleep with
happily married men.**

BRITT EKLUND
English model, actress

*For some people,
sex is so good it's scary.
Is that bad?
Let's be reasonable:
if sex is good, lots of sex
is even better.
Good sex can make you a
better person. So lots of sex might
make you the finest person
you can be.
Your body isn't just
your temple, it's also
your holy brothel.*

EURYDICE
American sex columnist

When women go wrong,
men go right after them.
MAE WEST (1893–1980)
American actress

A girl can wait for
the right man to come
along, but in the meantime
that still doesn't mean
she can't have a
wonderful time with
all the wrong ones.
CHER (B. 1946)
American actress

To the chagrin of my
inner slut, I'm just not
a very bad girl in real life.
In fact I'm almost too
good, and that may be
at the root of my fetish
for discipline, bringing
to light the short-skirted
infidel inside me,
letting her out for a
night or three.
CHRIS DALEY
American writer

What's the difference between a prostitute and a politician? There are some things a prostitute won't do for money.

NORMA JEAN ALMODOVAR (B. 1951)
American prostitute, writer and activist

A slut shares his sexuality
the way a philanthropist
shares her money—because
they have a lot of it to share,
because it makes them
happy to share it, because
sharing makes the world a
better place.
DOSSIE EASTON
American therapist and writer
CATHERINE A. LISZT
American writer and educator

*On favorite questions
he's been asked about sex:*
At a swing party,
I say it's bad etiquette
to be the first to take
out a whip. One should
wait for the host or
hostess to do so first.
Don't you agree?
DR. MARTY KLEIN
*American marriage counselor
and sex therapist*

Sex is the point of contact between man and nature, where morality and good intentions fall to primitive urges.

CAMILLE PAGLIA (B. 1947)
American author, critic, educator

You get a better class of person at orgies…. Everybody is very polite to each other. The conversation isn't very good, but you can't have everything.

GORE VIDAL (B. 1925)
American novelist, critic, and screenwriter

If God had meant us to have group sex, he'd have given us more organs.

MALCOLM BRADBURY (1932–2000)
British writer

Christianity gave Eros poison to drink; he did not die of it, but he degenerated into vice.

FRIEDRICH NIETZSCHE (1844–1900)
German philosopher

Threeways are so physically and emotionally exhausting because they do not occur in nature. You never see a gazelle threeway on a [*National Geographic*] special. Because they know better. Only man is fool enough to spit in the eye of God…God does not like threeways.

LISA CARVER (B. 1969)
American writer

Sex is natural, but not if it's done right.

ANONYMOUS

Those who restrain desire do so because theirs is weak enough to be restrained.

WILLIAM BLAKE (1757–1827)
British poet

Why should we take advice on sex from the Pope? If he knows anything about it, he shouldn't.

GEORGE BERNARD SHAW (1856–1950)
Irish playwright, critic

Those who restrain desire do so because theirs is weak enough to be restrained.

WILLIAM BLAKE (1757–1827)
British poet

I regret to say that we of the FBI are powerless to act in cases of oral-genital intimacy, unless it has in some way obstructed interstate commerce.

J. EDGAR HOOVER (1895–1972)
American FBI director

On the topic of faked orgasms, if sex fraud were a crime, I'd be in jail for the rest of my life.

MERRILL MARKOE
American writer, humorist

It is impossible to obtain a conviction for sodomy from an English jury. Half of them don't believe it can be physically done, and the other half are doing it.

WINSTON CHURCHILL (1874–1965)
British statesman

If homosexuality were normal, God would have created Adam and Bruce.

ANITA BRYANT (B. 1940)
American singer and writer

When authorities warn of the sinfulness of sex, there is an important lesson to be learned: do not have sex with the authorities.

MATT GROENING (B.1954)
American cartoonist

My mother said it was simple to keep a man; you must be a maid in the living room, a cook in the kitchen and a whore in the bedroom. I said I'd hire the other two and take care of the bedroom bit.

JERRY HALL (B. 1956)
American model

The Bible contains six admonishments to homosexuals and 362 admonishments to heterosexuals. That doesn't mean that God doesn't love heterosexuals. It's just that they need more supervision.

LYNN LAVNER
American comedian

If you can't be a good example, then you'll just have to be a horrible warning.

CATHERINE AIRD (B. 1930)
British writer

The old-fashioned girl yielded to a man's embraces as if she were lowering herself into a tub of cold water.

JAMES THURBER (1894–1961)
American writer, humorist

We are taught that man most loves and admires the domestic type of woman. This is one of the roaring jokes of history. The breakers of hearts, the queens of romance, the goddesses of a thousand devotees have not been cooks.

CHARLOTTE PERKINS GILMAN
(1860–1935)
American writer

The odds are usually 2:1 in favor of sex. You and she against her conscience.

EVAN ESAR (1899–1995)
American writer

I'll wager that in ten years it will be fashionable again to be a virgin.

BARBARA CARTLAND (1901–2000)
British romance novelist

Today's unspeakable perversion is tomorrow's kink, is next week's good clean fun.

DAN SAVAGE
American sex-advice columnist

The so-called new morality is the old immorality condoned.

LORD SHAWCROSS (B. 1902)
British lawyer, politician

If everything was coated with a seal of approval, some of the fun would go out of it. Let's get away with something. Degrade me, baby.

SALLIE TISDALE (B. 1957)
American writer

Sex is not sin. Many people have complained that this is taking all the fun out of sex.

DR. RUTH WESTHEIMER (B. 1928)
German-born American sex therapist and author

Christ died for our sins. Dare we make his martyrdom meaningless by not committing them?

JULES FEIFFER (B. 1929)
American cartoonist, writer

Should we all confess our sins to one another, we would all laugh at one another for our lack of originality.

KAHLIL GIBRAN (1883–1931)
Lebanese-Syrian philosopher

The first day of Spring was once the time for taking the young virgins into the fields, there in dalliance to set an example in fertility for nature to follow. Now we just set the clock an hour ahead and change the oil in the crankcase.

E. B. WHITE (1899–1985)
American writer

People's sex habits are as well known in Hollywood as their political opinions, and much less criticized.

BEN HECHT (1894–1964)
American journalist and writer

For a long time I was ashamed of the way I lived. I didn't reform. I'm just not ashamed anymore.

MAE WEST (1893–1980)
American actress

Abstinence is the mother of shameless lust.

PAT CALIFIA (B. 1959)
American writer, activist

No matter how many posters I hold up saying, "I'm a big pervert and I'm so happy about it," there's this part of me that's like, "How could I be this way?"

SUSIE BRIGHT (B. 1958)
American writer, editor

We may come to realize that chastity is no more a virtue than malnutrition.

DR. ALEX COMFORT (1920–2000)
British writer, sexologist

When "morality" is discussed I invariably discover, halfway into the conversation, that what is meant are not the great ethical questions…but the rather dreary business of sexual habit, which to my mind is an aesthetic rather than an ethical issue.

EDMUND WHITE (B. 1940)
American author

Lord, make me chaste— but not yet.

ST. AUGUSTINE (354–430)
Roman philosopher, scholar

Have you swallowed your husband's semen in the hope that because of your diabolical deed he might burn all the more with love and desire for you? If you have done this, you should do penance for seven years on legitimate holy days.

BURCHARD OF WORMS (C. 950–1025)
German bishop

Our American people are
a pretty homely and
wholesome crowd.
Cockeyed philosophies of life,
ugly sex situations,
cheap jokes and
dirty dialogue are not wanted.
Decent people
don't like this sort of stuff,
and it's our job
to see to it that they get
none of it.

JOSEPH BREEN
Code Enforcement Officer for the Motion Picture Association of America

WE OUGHT TO LOCATE OUR THINKING ABOUT SEXUALITY IN TERMS OF THE BEAUTY AND HOLINESS OF LIFE, NOT IN TERMS OF SOME REPRESSIVE SYSTEM BEING IMPOSED UPON LIFE.

JOHN SPONG (B. 1931)
American Episcopalian bishop, writer

Contempt of sexuality is a crime against life.

FRIEDRICH NIETZSCHE (1844–1900)
German philosopher

If a man is pictured chopping off a woman's breast, it only gets an R rating. But if, God forbid, a man is pictured kissing a woman's breast, it gets an X rating. Why is violence more acceptable than tenderness?

SALLY STRUTHERS (B. 1948)
American actress

A little coitus never hoitus.

ANONYMOUS

Let my lusts be my ruin then, for all else is fake and a mockery.

HART CRANE (1899–1932)
American poet

Eroticism has its own moral justifications because it says that pleasure is enough for me; it is a statement of the individual's sovereignty.

MARIO VARGAS-LLOSA (B. 1936)
Peruvian novelist, journalist

Sexual pleasure, wisely used and not abused, may prove the stimulus and liberator of our finest and most exalted activities.

HAVELOCK ELLIS (1859–1936)
British physician, writer

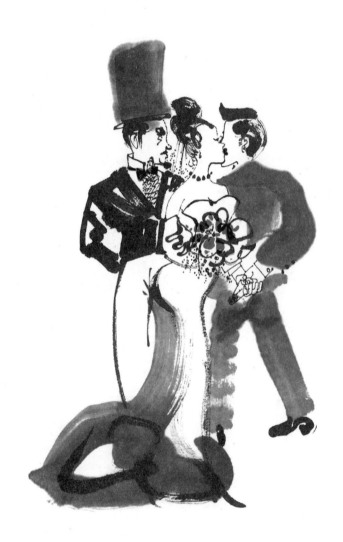

LOVE, RELATIONSHIPS, SEX: IS THREE A CROWD?

Just about everybody loves good sex.

But whether you can have good sex with

someone you love seems a matter of much dispute.

Love and sex should work well together, theoretically

speaking. But to hear men and women talk about

them is to listen to two very different subjects

discussed in very different languages. Perhaps

someday love, sex, men and women will all live

in harmony on the same side of the chasm.

Until then, we have only thoughts like these

to bridge the gap.

He said, "I can't remember when we last had sex," and I said, "well I can and that's why we ain't doing it."

ROSEANNE BARR (B. 1952)
American actress, comedian

Sex is the one thing you cannot really swindle…. Sex lashes out against counterfeit emotion, and is ruthless, devastating against false love.

D. H. LAWRENCE (1885–1930)
British author

One can learn technique, but never feeling…without love the most perfect technique is worthless and becomes merely a soulless artifice.

A. COSTLER M.D.
American physician

When one is pretending, the entire body revolts.

ANAIS NIN (1903–1977)
French writer

Sex without love is a s hollow and ridiculous as love without sex.

HUNTER S. THOMPSON (B. 1939)
American writer

When I look back on the pain of sex, the love like a wild fox so ready to bite, the antagonism that sits like a twin beside love, and contrast it with affection, so deeply unrepeatable, of two people who have lived a rich life together…it's the affection I find richer. It's that I would have again. Not all those doubtful rainbow colors.

ERIC BAGNOLD (1889–1981)
British novelist, playwright

To me the term "sexual freedom" meant freedom from having sex.

JANE WAGNER (B. 1935)
American writer, actress and director

Marriage is popular because it combines the maximum of temptation with the maximum of opportunity.

GEORGE BERNARD SHAW (1856–1950)
Irish playwright, critic

The best thing about being in a relationship is having someone right there to do it with when you're horny.

JENNY MCCARTHY (B. 1972)
American actress

The highest level of sexual excitement is in a monogamous relationship.

WARREN BEATTY (B. 1937)
American actor, director

Love is it's own aphrodisiac and is the main ingredient for lasting sex.

MORT KATZ (B. 1925)
American psychotherapist, writer

It's terrific to have a woman in your life who feeds the chickens while wearing one of your shirts, black underwear and stiletto heels.

PETER STRAUSS (B. 1947)
American actor

Love is not the dying moan of a distant violin. It's the triumphant twang of a bedspring.

S. J. PERLMAN (1904–1979)
American writer

Life in Lubbock, Texas taught me two things. One is that God loves you and you're going to burn in hell. The other is that sex is the most awful, filthy thing on earth. And you should save it for someone you love.

BUTCH HANCOCK (B. 1945)
American singer-songwriter

YOU CAN'T REMEMBER SEX...
THERE IS NO MEMORY OF IT IN THE BRAIN,
ONLY THE DEDUCTION THAT IT HAPPENED AND THAT
TIME PASSED, LEAVING YOU WITH A SILHOUETTE
THAT YOU WANT TO FILL IN AGAIN.

E. L. DOCTOROW (B. 1931)
American writer

Love is a fire.
But whether it is going to warm
your hearth or burn down your house,
you can never tell.

JOAN CRAWFORD (1906–1977)
American actress

There is a love that begins in the head and goes down to the heart, and grows slowly; but it lasts 'till death, and asks less than it gives. There is another love, that blots out wisdom, that is sweet with the sweetness of life and bitter with the bitterness of death, lasting for an hour, but it is worth having lived a whole life for that hour.

RALPH IRON (1855–1920)
South African writer

Sexuality is something, like nuclear energy, which may prove amenable to domestication…but then again, may not.

SUSAN SONTAG (B. 1933)
American writer

I know what I wish Ralph Nader would investigate next. Marriage. It's not safe. It's not safe at all.

JEAN KERR (B. 1923)
American playwright

Love is a snowmobile racing across the tundra and then suddenly it flips over, pinning you underneath. At night, the ice weasels come.

MATT GROENING (B.1954)
American cartoonist

Penguins mate for life. Which doesn't exactly surprise me that much 'cause they all look alike— it's not like they're gonna meet a better-looking penguin someday.

ELLEN DEGENERES (B. 1958)
American comedian

I don't breed well in
captivity.

GLORIA STEINEM (B. 1934)
American writer, editor

More extreme forms of
bondage involve homes in
the suburbs, station wagons,
household food budgets,
and Little League coaching
activities and are too alarm-
ing and repulsive to discuss
in print.

P. J. O'ROURKE (B. 1947)
American writer, editor

The bonds of wedlock are so heavy it takes two to carry them— sometimes three.

ALEXANDRE DUMAS (1802–1870)
French writer

You know of course that
the Tasmanians, who never
committed adultery, are
now extinct.

W. SOMERSET MAUGHAM (1874–1965)
British writer

Some people ask the
secret of our long marriage.
We take time to go
to a restaurant two times
a week. A little candlelight
dinner, music and dancing.
She goes Tuesdays,
I go Fridays.

HENNY YOUNGMAN (1906–1998)
American comedian

I haven't known any
open marriages although
quite a few have been ajar.

ZSA ZSA GABOR (B. 1919)
Hungarian-born American actress

I never married because
I have three pets at home
that answer the same
purpose as a husband.
I have a dog that growls
every morning, a parrot
that swears all afternoon,
and a cat that comes
home late at night.

MARIE CORELLI (1855–1924)
British writer

The love bird is one hundred percent faithful to his mate, as long as they are locked together in the same cage.

WILL CUPPY (1884–1949)
American humorist, journalist

My wife has cut our love-making down to once a month, but I know two guys she's cut out entirely.

RODNEY DANGERFIELD (B. 1922)
American comedian

After fifteen years of marriage, they finally achieved sexual compatibility. They both had a headache.

ANONYMOUS

My wife is a sex object—every time I ask for sex, she objects.

LES DAWSON (1934–1993)
British comedian

The only reason that I would take up jogging is so that I could hear heavy breathing again.

ERMA BOMBECK (1927–1996)
American humorist

Do you know what it means to come home at night to a woman who'll give you a little love, a little affection, a little tenderness? It means you're in the wrong house, that's what it means.

GEORGE BURNS (1896–1996)
American comedian

I know nothing about sex because I was always married.

ZSA ZSA GABOR (B. 1919)
Hungarian-born American actress

Sex drive—a physical craving begins in adolescence and ends at marriage.

ROBERT BYRNE (B. 1930)
American writer

Entering our lives' third quarter she'd been bored stiff with me and I bored limp with her....

JOHN BARTH (B. 1930)
American writer

Marriage, if it is to survive, must be treated as the beginning, not as the happy ending....

FEDERICO FELLINI (1920–1993)
Italian filmmaker

Some of you who have
already been around the block
may have dabbled
dangerously
in sexual pleasure. It's time
to straighten up and fly right.
You're a wife and
mother now—do you want
people to think you're some
disgusting slut?
If you don't have
a headache by now,
start sniffing
glue.

SUSIE BRIGHT (B. 1958)
American writer, editor

I AM HAPPY NOW THAT CHARLES CALLS
ON MY BEDCHAMBER LESS FREQUENTLY
THAN OF OLD. AS IT IS, I CAN ENDURE BUT TWO CALLS
A WEEK, AND WHEN I HEAR HIS FOOTSTEPS OUTSIDE
MY DOOR, I LIE DOWN ON MY BED, CLOSE MY EYES,
OPEN MY LEGS AND THINK OF ENGLAND.

ALICE LADY HILLDINGDON
(1857–1940)
English socialite

I've had it with the people who complain to the Advisor that their sex lives dwindle the longer they are with someone…. My husband and I sneak sex whenever we can. Our eight-year-old often can be heard telling the three-year-old, "Leave them alone, they will be done soon."

A. E. OF TEMECULA, CALIFORNIA
In a letter to Playboy

No chupa, no shtupa
(No wedding, no bedding).

YIDDISH PROVERB

The perfect lover is one who turns into a pizza at 4 a.m.

CHARLES PIERCE
American entertainer

We waste time looking for the perfect lover, instead of creating the perfect love.

TOM ROBBINS (B. 1936)
American writer

True love comes quietly, without banners or flashing lights. If you hear bells, get your ears checked.

ERICH SEGAL (B. 1937)
American writer

Any gal is gonna go out of her mind when she looks at her husband one day and realizes that she is not living with a man any longer. She is living with a reclining chair that burps.

ROSEANNE BARR (B. 1952)
American comedian

Men reach their sexual peak at eighteen. Women reach their sexual peak at thirty-five. Do you get the feeling God is into practical jokes? We're reaching our sexual peak right around the same time they're discovering they have a favorite chair.

RITA RUDNER (B. 1955)
American comedian

Marriage is the deep, deep peace of the double-bed after the hurly-burly of the chaise lounge.

MRS. PATRICK CAMPBELL (1865–1940)
English actress

Warning signs that your lover is bored.
1. Passionless kisses
2. Frequent sighing
3. Moved, left no
   forwarding address

MATT GROENING (B.1954)
American cartoonist

It is impossible to become bored in the presence of a mistress.

STENDHAL (1783–1842)
French writer

Sara could commit adultery at one end and weep for her sins at the other, and enjoy both operations at the same time.

JOYCE CARY (1888–1957)
Irish writer

On a man discovering his wife's infidelity:
Suddenly and ironically, she was becoming the kind of woman he had long idealized in his fantasies— the daring, carefree, sexually liberated woman he had searched for.

GAY TALESE (B. 1932)
American writer

Every man wants a woman to appeal to his better side, his nobler instincts and his higher nature—and another woman to help him forget them.

HELEN ROWLAND (1875–1950)
American journalist

*The happiest moment
of any affair takes place
after the loved one
has learned to accommodate
the lover and before
the maddening personality of
either party has emerged
like a jagged rock from
the receding tides
of lust and curiosity.*

QUENTIN CRISP (1908–1999)
British writer

There are women whose infidelities are the only link they have with their husbands.

SACHA GUITRY (1885–1957)
French writer, actor and film director

Darling, you're divine. I've had an affair with your husband. You'll be next.

TALLULAH BANKHEAD (1903–1968)
American actress

A man can have two, or maybe three love affairs while he is married. After that it is cheating.

YVES MONTAND (1921–1991)
French actor, singer

The first breath of adultery is the freest: after it, constraints aping marriage develop.

JOHN UPDIKE (B.1932)
American writer

There is only one real tragedy in a woman's life.
The fact that her past is always her lover,
and her future invariably her husband.

OSCAR WILDE (1854–1900)
Irish playwright

There is one thing I would break up over, and that is if she caught me with another woman. I won't stand for that.

STEVE MARTIN (B. 1945)
American comedian

Husbands are chiefly good lovers when they are betraying their wives.

MARILYN MONROE (1926–1962)
American actress

My wife's married. I'm not.

CHARLES BARKLEY (B. 1963)
American professional basketball player

A man can sleep around, no questions asked, but if a woman makes nineteen or twenty mistakes, she's a tramp.

JOAN RIVERS (B.1933)
American comedian

I just had a brief summer fling. I had a gay boyfriend and a straight boyfriend. We went on bike rides at midnight in the graveyards and it was very romantic.

MARGARET CHO (B. 1968)
American comedian

Love and sex can go together and sex and unlove can go together and love and unsex can go together. But personal love and personal sex is bad.

ANDY WARHOL (1928–1987)
American pop artist

I can understand companionship. I can understand bought sex in the afternoon. I cannot understand the love affair.

GORE VIDAL (B. 1925)
American writer, screenwriter

The zipless fuck is absolutely pure. It is free of ulterior motives. There is no power game. The man is not taking and the woman is not giving. No one is attempting to cuckold a husband or humiliate a wife. No one is trying to prove anything or get anything out of anyone. The zipless fuck is the purest thing there is. And it is rarer than the unicorn.

ERICA JONG (B. 1942)
American writer

Sex without love is an empty experience, but, as empty experiences go, it's one of the best.

WOODY ALLEN (B. 1935)
American filmmaker, actor and writer

The sex relation is not a personal relation. It can be irresistibly desired and rapturously consummated between persons who could not endure one an other for a day in any other relation.

GEORGE BERNARD SHAW
(1856–1950)
Irish playwright, critic

I've only been in love with a beer bottle and a mirror.

SID VICIOUS (1957–1979)
British musician

Couples have to liberate
masturbation, accept
self-pleasuring in each other,
show one another how
to do it. And if a man can't
handle seeing his lover
use a vibrator, my advice
to the woman is: keep
the vibrator and recycle
the man.

BETTY DODSON (B. 1929)
American sexuality guru

Don't knock masturbation—
it's sex with someone I love.

WOODY ALLEN (B. 1935)
American filmmaker, writer and actor

At the end, Schwarzenegger
makes his ritual preparations
for the climactic showdown,
decking himself out in
leather, packing up an
arsenal of guns, and,
as he leaves the apartment,
copping a quick look of
satisfaction in the mirror.
It's his only love scene.

PAULINE KAEL (1919–1991)
American film critic

When you look back at
your life…what you really
find out is that the only
person you really go to
bed with is yourself.

SHIRLEY MACLAINE (B. 1934)
American actress, writer

59

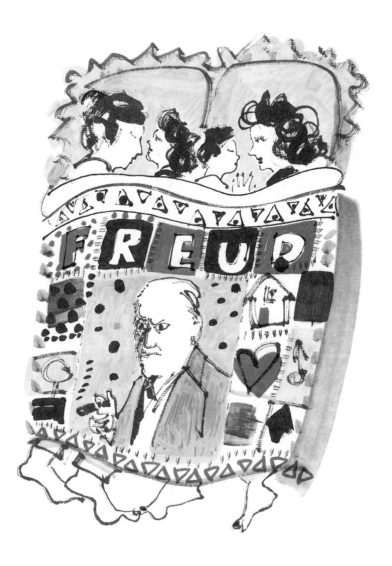

SEX ON THE BRAIN

Contrary to morning-after alibis, the brain does

almost all of the thinking in sexual matters.

Our minds serve as instigators, judges, diplomats,

entertainers, critics, matchmakers, psychologists

and creative directors for our loins.

Still, the relationship isn't an entirely happy

or stable one. So our brains have also ordered

our mouths to offer up explanations like these.

Pleasure is the object,
the duty, the goal
Of all rational creatures.

VOLTAIRE (1694–1778)
French writer, philosopher

Last time I tried to
make love to my wife,
nothing was happening,
so I said to her,
"What's the matter?
You can't think of
anybody either?"

RODNEY DANGERFIELD (B. 1922)
American comedian

A man and his partner
had this elaborate sexual
fantasy they were trying
to make a reality.
They wanted to make a
wall-to-wall, room-size
pizza. He'd dress up as
a garlic clove and she'd
dress up as a pepperoni.
With classical music
playing in the background,
they'd run across the
room, meet in the
middle and start

**Phebe: Good shepherd, tell this
youth what 'tis to love.
Silvius: It is to be all made of fantasy.**

FROM WILLIAM SHAKESPEARE'S
AS YOU LIKE IT

When turkeys mate
they think of swans.

JOHNNY CARSON (B. 1925)
American television host

During sex, I fantasize
that I'm someone else.

RICHARD LEWIS (B. 1947)
American comedian

coupling. They wanted
to know if the oil
on the pizza would
weaken their
condom.

ISADORA ALMAN
American therapist and sex columnist

An improper mind
is a perpetual feast.

LOGAN PEARSALL SMITH (1881–1943)
American writer

Sex is our deepest
form of consciousness.
It is utterly non-ideal,
non-mental.
It is pure blood-consciousness....
It is the consciousness
of the night, when
the soul is
almost asleep.

D. H. LAWRENCE (1885–1930)
British writer

You are what you dream.
You are what you daydream.
Masters and Johnson's charts and
numbers and flashing lights and plastic
pricks tell us everything about sex
and nothing about it.
Because sex is all in the head.

ERICA JONG (B. 1942)
American writer

The mind I love must have
wild places, a tangle orchard
where dark damsons drop
in the heavy grass, an
overgrown little wood,
the chance of a snake or
two, a pool that nobody's
fathomed the depth of,
and paths threaded
with flowers planted
by the mind.

KATHERINE MANSFIELD (1888–1923)
New Zealand-born British author

We English have sex on the
brain, which is not the most
satisfactory place for it.

MALCOLM MUGGERIDGE (1903–1990)
British writer

A great portion [of semen]
cometh from the brain.

AMBROSE PARE
16th-century French physician

I think I have a dick
in my brain. I don't need
one between my legs.

MADONNA (B. 1958)
American pop star

**I have a brain and
a uterus, and I use
them both.**

PATRICIA SCHROEDER (B. 1940)
American congresswoman

See, the problem is that God gives men a brain and a penis, and only enough blood to run one at a time.

ROBIN WILLIAMS (B. 1952)
American comedian, actor

Isn't it interesting how the sounds are the same for an awful nightmare and great sex?

RUE MCCLANAHAN (B. 1935)
American actress

If it is not erotic, it is not interesting.

FERNANDO ARRABAL (B. 1932)
Spanish writer

An intellectual is someone who has found something more interesting than sex.

EDGAR WALLACE (1875–1932)
British writer

Once a philosopher, twice a pervert.

VOLTAIRE (1694–1778)
French writer, philosopher

Philosophy is to the real world what masturbation is to sex.

KARL MARX (1818–1883)
German philosopher, economist

Masturbation is the thinking man's television.

CHRISTOPHER HAMPTON (B. 1946)
British writer

There are no chaste minds. Minds copulate wherever they meet.

ERIC HOFFER (1902–1983)
American writer

In my sex fantasy, nobody ever loves me for my mind.

NORA EPHRON (B. 1941)
American writer, screenwriter

65

Men aren't attracted to me by my mind. They're attracted to me by what I don't mind.

GYPSY ROSE LEE (1914–1970)
American actress, burlesque stripper

THEY THINK THEY'RE GOING TO GET
ONLINE AND TYPE DIRTY WORDS AND
MASTURBATE, BUT MANY PEOPLE
FIND THEMSELVES FALLING IN LOVE...
FOR MEN AND WOMEN
WHO DON'T HAVE THAT KIND OF SEXUAL
CANDOR IN THEIR LIVES—WHO NEVER
HAD THAT FREEDOM TO EXPRESS
THEMSELVES—WHEN THEY FIND
SOMEONE THEY CAN DO THAT WITH,
IT'S A HEAVY CONNECTION.

LISA PALAC (B. 1963)
American writer, editor

When you sleep with someone you take off a lot more than your clothes.

ANNA QUINDLEN (B. 1952)
American journalist

Stripping's not so much about your body as it is about tapping into your sexual power. If I were a therapist, I'd say, "Jane, I know you're tired, you're

There's nothing wrong with a person's sex life that the right psychoanalyst can't exaggerate.

GERALD HORTON BATH

I love her, too, but our neuroses just don't match.

ARTHUR MILLER (B. 1915)
American playwright

Love is two minutes, fifty-two seconds of squishing noises. It shows your mind isn't clicking right.

JOHN LYDON (A.K.A. JOHNNY ROTTEN) (B. 1956)
British musician

---

feeling like your husband doesn't desire you. But down at the Star Guard, they have an amateur night on Monday and they pay $500. Get up there, do it!"

KARI WUHRER (B. 1967)
American actress

Love is a grave mental illness.

PLATO
Greek philosopher (427–347 B.C.)

There is always some madness in love, but there is always some reason in madness.

FRIEDRICH NIETZSCHE (1844–1900)
German philosopher

The only time human beings are sane is the ten minutes after intercourse.

ERIC BERNE (1910–1970)
American psychiatrist

67

Reason doesn't just leave us when we enter an orgasm; orgasm is antithetical to reason— orgasm destroys reason and, conversely, a moment of reason can destroy an orgasm.

SALLY TISDALE (B. 1957)
American writer

I'm a bad lover.
I once caught a peeping Tom booing me.

RODNEY DANGERFIELD (B. 1922)
American comedian

I'm not much interested in why it is that I find glasses on women sexy.... Sensual pleasure—any kind of pleasure—calls out to be savored more than explained.

CHARLES TAYLOR
American writer

When beauty fires the blood, how love exalts the mind!

JOHN DRYDEN (1631–1700)
British poet

Beauty isn't everything!
But then what is?

LANFORD WILSON (B. 1937)
American playwright

I'm tired of all this nonsense about beauty being only skin deep. That's deep enough. What do you want— an adorable pancreas?

JEAN KERR (B. 1923)
American playwright

The most common error made in matters of appearance is the belief that one should disdain the superficial and let the true beauty of one's soul shine through. If there are places on your body where this is a possibility, you are not attractive—you are leaking.

FRAN LEBOWITZ (B. 1951)
American writer, humorist

Some people have flat feet. Some people have dandruff. I have this appalling imagination.

TOM EWELL (1909–1994)
American actor

A little theory makes
sex more interesting,
more comprehensible, and
less scary—too much
is a put-down, especially
as you're likely to get it out
of perspective and become
a spectator of your own
performance.

DR. ALEX COMFORT (1920–2000)
British writer, sexologist

Sex is not imaginary,
but it is not quite real either.

MASON COOLEY (B. 1927)
American aphorist.

My ultimate fantasy
is to entice a man to
my bedroom, put a gun
to his head and say,
"Make babies or die."

RUBY WAX
American-born British actress,
comedian and writer

If the world were a
different place, a happy
rainbow place filled with
total peace and harmony,
maybe then I would come
all the time from thinking
about making love in a
field of daisies.

LISA PALAC (B. 1963)
American writer, editor

We think about sex
obsessively except
during the act, when our
minds tend to wander.

HOWARD NEMEROV (B. 1920)
American poet

I don't think when
I make love.

BRIGITTE BARDOT (B. 1934)
French actress

To think is to say no.

EMILE CHARTIER (1868–1951)
French writer

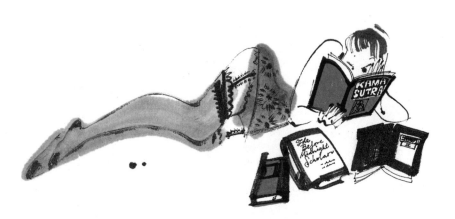

SEX ED.: LEARNING THE GROPES

These days, undergraduate degrees in "the birds
and the bees" are awarded by a variety of instructors
and learning institutions, including sitcom writers,
school playground know-it-alls, Internet chat rooms,
magazines, and a seemingly endless faculty of "sexperts."
Some of these are not necessarily bad places to get
started in learning about sex. But work on your
Masters in Sexual Practice can — and should —
take a lifetime of learning and involve material
from as many credible sources as you can get
your hands on. Here's some credible, not-so-credible,
and incredible sources to thumb through.

From bestsellers to comic books, any child who hasn't acquired an extensive sex education by the age of 12 belongs in remedial reading.

WILL STANTON (B. 1918)
American writer

Sex is hereditary.
If your parents never
had it, chances are
you won't either.

MURPHY'S LAW

I only have two rules
for my newly born daughter:
she will dress well and
never have sex.

JOHN MALKOVICH (B. 1953)
American actor

Before the child ever
gets to school it will have
received crucial, almost
irrevocable sex education
and this will have been
taught by the parents,
who are not aware of
what they are doing.

DR. MARY S. CALDERONE (1904–1998)
American physician, writer

Don't bother discussing sex
with small children. They
rarely have anything to add.

FRAN LEBOWITZ (B. 1951)
American writer, humorist

**If my teacher could
have influenced
my sexuality,
I would have turned
out to be a nun.**

GEORGE CARLIN (B. 1937)
American comedian

Who could have
supposed that this
childish punishment,
received at the age of
eight at the hands of a
woman of thirty, would
determine my tastes and
desires, my passions,
my very self for the
rest of my life.

JEAN-JACQUES ROUSSEAU (1712–1778)
French philosopher

My favorite book
when I was eight was
*Everything You Always
Wanted to Know About
Sex—But Were Afraid to
Ask.* I was not afraid to ask.
DREW BARRYMORE (B. 1975)
American actress

*On accelerating teen
promiscuity:*
I see girls, seventh and
eighth graders, even sixth
graders, who tell me they're
virgins, and they're going
to wait to have intercourse
until they meet the man
they'll marry. But then
they've had oral sex fifty
or sixty times.
PSYCHOLOGIST DR. WAYNE WARREN
From the New York Times

There is nothing like
early promiscuous sex
for dispelling life's bright
mysterious expectations.
IRIS MURDOCH (1919–1999)
British writer

The first time we ever
made love I said,
"Am I the first man who
ever made love to you?"
She said, "You could be.
You look damn familiar."
RONNIE BULLARD
American comedian

I wouldn't like
to sleep with a guy
who was a virgin.
I'd have to teach him
stuff and I don't
have the patience.
MADONNA (B. 1957)
American pop star

No one is more carnal
than a recent virgin.
JOHN STEINBECK (1902–1968)
American writer

Nature abhors a virgin—
a frozen asset.
CLARE BOOTHE LUCE (1903–1987)
American playwright, ambassador

**I didn't want it like that.
Not against the bricks or hunkering in
somebody's car. I wanted it to come undone
like a gold thread, like a tent full of birds.**
SANDRA CISNEROS (B. 1954)
American writer

SEX ED.: LEARNING THE GROPES

I DO GIVE A GOOD BLOW JOB.
I REALLY, REALLY DO,
AND I WISH YOU COULD GET
A GRADE, OR SOME TYPE
OF CERTIFICATE.
I REALIZED I WAS REALLY
GOOD AT IT, I GUESS,
WHEN I WAS 20 OR 21
YEARS OLD. I WAS GIVING
THIS GUY A BLOW JOB,
AND HE SAID,
"YOU DO THIS SO WELL.
WHAT ARE YOU
GOING TO DO WITH THE
REST OF YOUR LIFE?"

ELLEN CLEGHORNE (B. 1965)
American comedian

I kissed my first girl and smoked my first cigarette on the same day. I haven't had time for tobacco since.

ARTURO TOSCANINI (1867–1957)
Italian conductor

I think that if I had not had a previous relationship with a married man, I don't think the notion of having a relationship with the President would have been familiar to me.

MONICA LEWINSKY (B. 1973)
Former White House intern

Sex education is legitimate in that girls cannot be taught soon enough how children don't come into the world.

KARL KRAUS (1874–1936)
Austrian writer

Be wary of puppy love; it can lead to a dog's life.

GLADIOLA MONTANA
American humorist

Wanton kittens make sober cats.

ENGLISH PROVERB

I married the first man I ever kissed. When I tell my children that, they just about throw up.

BARBARA BUSH (B. 1925)
American first lady

"You kids think you invented sex," my mother was fond of saying. But hadn't we? With no instruction manual or federally-enforced training period, didn't we all come away feeling we'd discovered something unspeakably modern?

DAVID SEDARIS (B. 1957)
American writer, radio commentator

Women who miscalculate are called "mothers."

ABIGAIL VAN BUREN (1918–2002)
American advice columnist

Given a choice between hearing my daughter say "I'm pregnant" or "I used a condom," most mothers would get up in the middle of the night and buy them herself.

JOCELYN ELDERS (B. 1933)
American surgeon general

SEX ED.: LEARNING THE GROPES

Fewer college-age students today know the physiology of sex, and they depend much more on religious superstition and urban legend. They may know all about Britney Spears' belly button, but they wouldn't know the mechanics of a female orgasm if it popped out of their TV Screens.

SUSIE BRIGHT (B. 1958)
American writer, editor

Where do babies come from? Don't bother asking adults. They lie like pigs. However, diligent independent research and hours of playground consultation have yielded fruitful, if tentative, results. There are several theories. Near as we can figure out, it has something to do with acting ridiculous in the dark. We believe it is similar to dogs when they act peculiar and

---

On a college paper she wrote on masturbation: The research was remarkable!

CLAIRE DANES (B. 1979)
American actress

So many guys who can assemble a refrigerator for you, guys who can take apart your computer and put it back together again, guys who can fix your dishwasher, have no idea where anything is on a woman. Why can't we just give everyone, when we meet them, some sort of a manual, like you would when you buy a Cuisinart?

MERRILL MARKOE
American writer, humorist

ride each other. This is called "making love." Careful study of popular song lyrics, advertising catch-lines, TV sitcoms, movies, and T-Shirt inscriptions offers us significant clues as to its nature. Apparently it makes grown-ups insipid and insane. Some graffiti was once observed that said "sex is good." All available evidence, however, points to the contrary.

MATT GROENING (B. 1954)
American cartoonist

If our sex life were determined by our first youthful experiments, most of the world would be doomed to celibacy. In no area of human experience are human beings more convinced that something better can be had if only they persevere.

P. D. JAMES (B. 1920)
British writer

The day after that wedding night,
I found that a distance of a thousand
miles, abyss and discovery and
irremediable metamorphosis,
separated me from the day before.

COLETTE
French writer

A woman has got
to love a bad man once
or twice in her life, to be
thankful for a good one.

MARJORIE KINNAN RAWLINGS
(1896–1953)
American writer

Sexual knowledge is
sexual knowledge,
and one way you learn
it is when you do it.
And most people haven't
done it as much as I have.

NINA HARTLEY (B. 1961)
American porn star

**These days, the
honeymoon is
rehearsed much
more often than
the wedding.**

P. J. O'ROURKE (B. 1947)
American writer, editor

I blame my mother
for my poor sex life.
All she told me was, "the
man goes on top and the
woman underneath."
For three years my husband
and I slept on bunk beds.

JOAN RIVERS (B. 1933)
American comedian

Women over thirty are
at their best, but men
over thirty are too old
to recognize it.

JEAN-PAUL BELMONDO (B. 1933)
French actor

The lovely thing about
being forty is that you
can appreciate twenty-five
year-old men more.

COLLEEN MCCULLOUGH (B. 1938)
Australian neurophysiologist and novelist

1. Get into bed upside down.
2. Never ask if it's in yet.
3. A man who can't kiss can't fuck.
4. No matter what he says, deep throating does not exist.
5. Never, ever go to bed with a man on the first date. Not ever. Unless you really want to.
6. Baby talk is not an aphrodisiac.
7. No whips and handcuffs before the third date.
8. If you suck on his fingers, you'd better not be kidding.
9. Oral sex is a great way to tone up your cheekbones.
10. Fondling a man's privates is not like testing peaches in the supermarket.

CYNTHIA HEIMEL
American writer, humorist

I used to be Snow White, but I drifted.

MAE WEST (1893–1980)
American actress

I'm as pure as the driven slush.

TALLULAH BANKHEAD (1903–1965)
American actress

Middle age dawns with the recognition that sex has become a relatively dull and dangerous waste of time—and that you'll never find anything better.

RUTH MARCOZZI (B. 1951)
American advice columnist

The best proof that experience is useless is that the end of one love does not disgust us from beginning another.

PAUL BOURGET (1852–1935)
French writer

I like men who have a future and women who have a past.

OSCAR WILDE (1854–1900)
Irish playwright

One day she was
sitting on the porch and
I said, "Granny, how old
does a woman get
before she don't want
no more boyfriends?"
(She was around 106 then.)
She said, "I don't know Honey.
You have to ask someone
older than me."

JACKIE "MOMS" MABLEY (1894–1975)
American comedian

Experience is the name everybody gives to their mistakes.

OSCAR WILDE (1854–1900)
Irish playwright

If I had my life to live over again, I'd make the same mistakes, only sooner.

TALLULAH BANKHEAD (1903–1965)
American actress

Honest women are inconsolable for the mistakes they haven't made.

SACHA GUITRY (1885–1957)
French writer, actor and film director

Quite a few women told me, one way or another, that they thought it was sex, not youth, that's wasted on the young....

JEAN HARRIS (B. 1923)
American writer

Too chaste an adolescence makes for a dissolute old age.

ANDRE GIDE (1869–1951)
French writer

If the young only knew; if the old only could.

FRENCH PROVERB

Sins become more subtle as you grow older: you commit sins of despair rather than lust.

PIERS PAUL READ (B. 1941)
British writer

Young men want to be faithful, and are not; old men want to be faithless, and cannot.

OSCAR WILDE (1854–1900)
Irish playwright

It's so hard for an old rake to turn over a new leaf.

JOHN BARRYMORE (1882–1942)
American actor

There is much to be said for post-menopausal celibacy.... No more diets to stay slim and desirable: I've had sex and I've had food, and I'd rather eat.

FLORENCE KING (B. 1936)
American humorist, essayist and social critic

I'm at the age where food has taken the place of sex in my life. In fact, I've just had a mirror put over my kitchen table.

RODNEY DANGERFIELD (B. 1922)
American comedian

If I felt any better, I'd be flying. I don't need Viagra. I need the opposite, man. I'm hornier than a toad.

JACK LALANNE AT AGE 85 (B. 1914)
American fitness pioneer

Sex after ninety is like trying to shoot pool with a rope. Even putting my cigar in its holder is a thrill.

GEORGE BURNS (1896–1996)
American comedian

It's ill-becoming for an old broad to sing about how bad she wants it. But occasionally we do.

LENA HORNE (B. 1917)
American singer, actress

The real fountain of youth is to have a dirty mind.

JERRY HALL (B. 1956)
American model

I feel that the older I get, the more shameless I feel. And in a sense, more pure.

MARIA IRENE FORNES (B. 1930)
American playwright

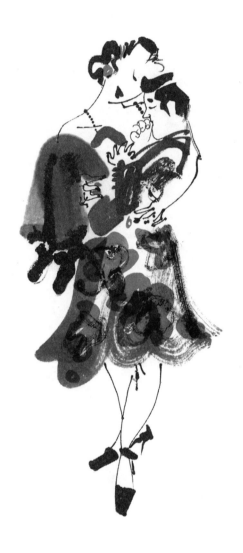

MEN AND WOMEN

The War Between the Sexes goes from toe-to-toe combat to groin-to-groin diplomacy, then back again. Despite the never-ending cycle of fighting and negotiation, the warriors still take time out to talk trash, assess, and praise their opponents on the other side of the gender line. Well, mostly to talk trash.

When a man says, "I'm no good at relationships. I have been alone for so long, perhaps I was meant to be alone!" or "You'll probably come to hate me, deep down I'm a real asshole," take him at his word and run like the wind!

CASSANDRA O'KEEFE
American writer, actress and artist

Make war, not love.
It's safer.

HENNY YOUNGMAN (1906–1998)
American comedian

Madame, shall we undress you for the fight?
The wars are naked that we make tonight.

GEORGE MOORE (1852–1933)
Irish novelist, poet and playwright

After making love I said to my girl, "Was it good for you, too?" And she said, "I don't think this was good for anybody."

GARY SHANDLING (B. 1949)
American comedian, writer and actor

The man who gets on best with women is the one who knows best how to get on without them.

CHARLES BAUDELAIRE (1821–1867)
French writer

I have come to think of orgasms as the things that I have really quickly while the guy gets up to look in the refrigerator for something to drink.

MERRILL MARKOE
American writer, humorist

If men knew what women laughed about, they would never sleep with us.

ERICA JONG (B. 1942)
American writer

I have always been principally interested in men for sex. I've always thought any sane woman would be a lover of women because loving men is such a mess. I have always wished I'd fall in love with a woman. Damn.

GERMAINE GREER (B. 1939)
Australian feminist, writer

I know a lot of women who use men, but the world is not perfect. Fifty years ago there was Hitler, now there are bitches everywhere.

JULIE DELPY (B. 1969)
French actress

Some women blush when they are kissed; some call for the police; some swear; some bite; but the worst are those who laugh.

ANONYMOUS

We all know men commit more violent acts. But they're not the ones [thinking] about cruelty. It's we women who pinch the sheets at 3 a.m., contemplating injustice and plotting revenge.

LISA CARVER (B. 1969)
American writer

On cutting off her husband's penis:
He always has an orgasm and he doesn't wait for me. He's selfish. I don't think it's fair, so I pulled back the sheets then, and I did it.

LORENA BOBBITT
Columbian-American housewife

Happy in love, Adam would have spared us history.

E. M. CIORAN (1911–1995)
Romanian philosopher

Women's orgasms are Mother Nature's way of conning heterosexual women into bedding down with men, thereby risking disease, pregnancy and conversations about pro sports.

DAN SAVAGE
American sex-advice columnist

*Ever since Adam, men
have rolled over onto
their side of the bed,
lit a cigarette, and asked,
"what were you thinking about?"
And the woman
has answered, "Nothing."
Or the more outspoken,
"You." How can men
have really believed
them all this time?*

NANCY FRIDAY (B. 1937)
American writer

When Eve saw her reflection in a pool, she sought Adam and accused him of infidelity.

AMBROSE BIERCE (1842–1914)
American writer, critic

Adultery may or may not be sinful, but it is never cheap.

RAYMOND POSTGATE (1896–1971)
British writer and historian

If you want to read about love and marriage, you've got to buy two separate books.

ALAN KING (B. 1924)
American comedian

The majority of husbands remind me of an orangutan trying to play the violin.

HONORE DE BALZAC (1799–1850)
French writer

The next time I have the urge to get married, I'm just going to find a woman I don't like and buy her a house.

LEWIS GRIZZARD (1946–1994)
American writer

Ah, yes, divorce— from the Latin word meaning to rip out a man's genitals through his wallet.

ROBIN WILLIAMS (B. 1952)
American comedian, actor

There's very little advice in men's magazines, because men don't think there's a lot they don't know. Women do. Women want to learn. Men think, "I know what I'm doing, just show me somebody naked."

JERRY SEINFELD (B. 1954)
American comedian

Have you heard of this new book entitled *1,001 Sex Secrets Men Should Know?* It contains comments from 1,001 women on how men can be better in bed. I think that women would actually settle for three: slow down, turn off the TV, call out the right name.

JAY LENO (B. 1950)
American television host

EASY SEX, WHERE A WOMAN LIES
ON A BED AND YOU GET ON TOP OF HER,
ISN'T VERY INTERESTING. I'M A MAN,
I LIKE A STRUGGLE, A CONQUEST.
I JUST HAPPEN TO LIKE BEING
THE LOSER, AND THEN MADE TO SATISFY
THE FEMALE WINNER.

ERIC STANTON (1926–1999)
American erotic cartoonist

Guys would sleep with a bicycle if it had the right color lip gloss on. They have no shame. They're like bull elks in a field. It's a scent to them, a smell.

TORI AMOS (B. 1963)
American musician

If you put a guy on a desert island, he'd do it to mud. A girl doesn't understand this: "You'd do it to mud—you don't love me!" Sex is a different emotion for women.

LENNY BRUCE (1925–1966)
American comedian

I love men. I think that's confusing for people. Like how could you be a dominatrix and beat men up…and like men. The thing is, exactly the opposite is true: if you don't like men, you'll never survive in this business.

MISTRESS NATASHA
American professional dominatrix

I love men, even though they're lyin', cheatin' scumbags.

GWYNETH PALTROW (B. 1972)
American actress

Being in touch with our inner Bitch ensures that we will have orgasms.

ELIZABETH HILTS
American writer

My advice is to look
to the bigger picture:
by expressing devotion
to one woman you
are setting yourself up
in very good graces
to the queen bee. And her
rewards are historically
proven to be far more
sensuous than a quick lay.

THURSTON MOORE (B. 1958)
American musician

Sex hasn't been the same since women started to enjoy it.

LEWIS GRIZZARD (1946–1994)
American writer

Straight men need
to be emasculated.
I'm sorry. They all need
to be slapped around.
Women have been kept
down for too long.

MADONNA (B. 1958)
American pop star

You have to accept
the fact that part
of the sizzle of sex
comes from the danger
of sex. You can be
overpowered.

CAMILLE PAGLIA (B. 1947)
American author, critic and educator

Sex used to be our most powerful
weapon against men. Not anymore.
Not since they found out we like it.
We lost a big one there.
Women aren't faking orgasms
anymore. They're hiding them.
"I didn't feel anything. Oh that?
That was the hiccups."

DIANE NICHOLS
American comedian

The big mistake that men
make is when they turn
thirteen or fourteen and
all of a sudden they've reached
puberty, they believe that
they like women.
Actually, you're just horny.
It doesn't mean you like
women any more at
twenty-one than you
did at ten.

JULES FEIFFER (B. 1929)
American cartoonist

A woman once asked me, "How can I get over my sexual obsession with gangsters?" She was only orgasmic with men who were dangerous. I told her to get her thrills elsewhere, like from deep-sea divers, Navy Seals or bungee jumpers. There has to be a better way to have an orgasm than collecting thugs.

PEPPER SCHWARTZ (B. 1945)
American therapist, author

Even though I got liberated, it's still very complicated. I say to men, "Okay, pretend you're a burglar and you've broken in here and you throw me down on the bed and make me suck your cock!" And they're horrified. It goes against all they've recently been taught. "No, no, it would degrade you!" Exactly. Degrade me when I ask you to.

LISA PALAC (B. 1963)
American writer, editor

People call me a feminist whenever I express sentiments that differentiate me from a doormat or a prostitute.

REBECCA WEST (1892–1983)
British writer, critic

Physically, the woman in intercourse is a space inhabited, a literal territory occupied literally: occupied even if there has been no resistance, no force; even if the occupied person said yes please, yes hurry, yes more.

ANDREA DWORKIN (B. 1946)
American feminist writer

Men who cherish for women the highest respect are seldom popular with them.

ANONYMOUS

I don't have the time every day to put on makeup. I need that time to clean my rifle.

HENRIETTE MANTEL
American actress, writer

We love our lipstick, have a passion for polish, and, basically, adore this armor that we call "fashion." To us, it's fun, it's feminine, and, in the particular way we flaunt it, it's definitely feminist.

DEBBIE STOLLER
American writer

I don't know one woman out there who doesn't want to feel strong and beautiful, dress up in fun costumes and tell somebody to go take a hike.

JOANIE LAURER (B. 1970)
American professional wrestler

There is a little bit of vampire instinct in every woman.

THEDA BARA (1890–1955)
American silent film star

What did one lesbian vampire say to the other? "See you next month."

ANONYMOUS

Women complain about Premenstrual Syndrome. But I think of it as the only time of the month I can be myself.

ROSEANNE BARR (B. 1952)
American comedian, actress

Men may love women, but they are in a rage with them, too. I believe it is a triumph of the human psyche that out of this contradiction, a new form of emotion emerges, one so human it is unknown to animals even one step lower in the evolutionary scale: passion.

NANCY FRIDAY (B. 1937)
American writer

The young women who grew up in Ms. households feel the need to assert that they're not anti-male, not anti-sex, that they don't believe all sex is rape. But they're also nobody's victim. There are two parts to these young women's view: One, they're going to enjoy sex; two, on their terms.

PATRICIA IRELAND (B. 1945)
American feminist

To me, sex wasn't an everyday thing. Attached to the woman's cunt was always the woman herself. The woman was the most interesting thing.

HENRY MILLER (1891–1980)
American writer

For he (Henry Miller) captured something in the sexuality of men as it had never been seen before, precisely that it was man's sense of awe before women, his dread of her position one step closer to eternity (for in that step were her powers) which made men detest women, revile them, humiliate them, defecate symbolically upon them, do everything to reduce them so that one might dare to enter them and take pleasure of them.

NORMAN MAILER (B. 1923)
American writer

Testosterone does not have to be toxic.

ANNA QUINDLEN (B. 1952)
American journalist, author

A hard man is good to find.

MAE WEST (1893–1980)
American actress

To be happy with a man you must understand him a lot and love him a little. To be happy with a woman you must love her a lot and not try to understand her at all.

HELEN ROWLAND (1875–1950)
American journalist

If all we have to choose from is the limp dick or the superhard dick, we're in trouble. We need a versatile dick who admits that intercourse isn't all there is to sexuality, who can negotiate rough sex on Monday, eating pussy on Tuesday and cuddling on Wednesday.

BELL HOOKS (B. 1952)
American writer

woman is. She remains in that precise place within man where darkness begins.

FEDERICO FELLINI (1920–1993)
Italian filmmaker

I refuse to consign the whole male sex to the nursery. I insist on believing that some men are my equals.

BRIGID BROPHY (1929–1995)
English writer

Men and women do little else but make trouble for each other, yet if a high wall separated them they would break it down to get through.

ED HOWE (1853–1937)
American journalist and humorist

Particularly for us Catholics, woman is seen as either the spirit or the flesh, as either the embodiment of virtue, motherhood and saintliness or the incarnation of vice, whoredom and wickedness…. The problem is to find the link between these opposites. But that is difficult, because we don't really know who

I'll do anything to pass the ERA [Equal Rights Amendment], even if it means wearing babydoll nightgowns and padded bras, if that will make people less afraid.

JOAN HACKETT (1934–1983),
American actress

What would men be without women? Scarce, sir, mighty scarce.

MARK TWAIN (1835–1910)
American humorist

The relation of
man to woman
is the flowing of
two rivers side by side,
sometimes mingling, then
separating again, and
traveling on.
The relationship
is a life-long change
and a life-long
traveling.

D. H. LAWRENCE (1885–1930)
British writer

Both men and women are bisexual in the psychological sense; I shall conclude that you have decided in your own minds to make "active" coincide with "masculine' and "passive" with "feminine." But I advise you against it.

SIGMUND FREUD (1856–1939)
Austrian physician and psychologist

There is more difference within the sexes than between them.

DAME IVY COMPTON-BURNETT (1884–1969)
English writer

The two sexes mutually corrupt and improve each another.

MARY WOLLSTONECRAFT (1759–1797)
English feminist, writer

Nobody will ever win the battle of the sexes. There's too much fraternizing with the enemy.

HENRY KISSINGER (B. 1923)
German-born American secretary of state

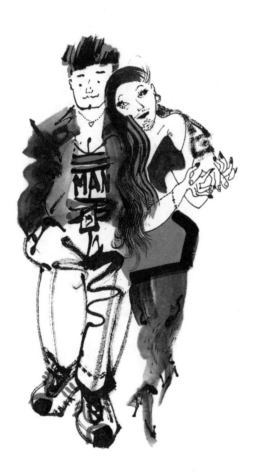

ALTERNATIVES

Pleasure is every bit as big a mother

as necessity when it comes to invention.

Those seeking sexual satisfaction have concocted —

and continue to concoct — a vast catalog

of new ways to tickle their fancies and rock

their worlds. Fortunately, rumor, gossip and

vivid description have remained just as ambitious

in keeping tabs on the developments.

There is no norm in sex. Norm is the name of a guy who lives in Brooklyn.

DR. ALEX COMFORT (1920–2000)
British writer, sexologist

There is hardly anyone whose sexual life, if it were broadcast, would not fill the world at large with surprise and horror.

W. SOMERSET MAUGHAM (1874–1965)
British writer

I'm not kinky, but occasionally I like to put on a robe and stand in front of a tennis ball machine.

GARY SHANDLING (B. 1949)
American comedian, writer and actor

Being kinky and single can be tough on the ego.

DR. GLORIA G. BRAME (B. 1955)
American writer

I enjoy dating married men because they don't want anything kinky, like breakfast.

JONI RODGERS (B. 1962)
American writer

Face it. After Marv Albert, no fetish is really shocking.

MAXIM MAGAZINE

Nothing risque, nothing gained.

ALEXANDER WOOLLCOTT
(1887–1943)
American writer

I'll try anything twice.

YANCY BUTLER
American actress

She was so wild that when she made French toast she got her tongue caught in the toaster.

RODNEY DANGERFIELD (B. 1922)
American comedian

Chocolate for me is just like an orgasm.

BRITNEY SPEARS (B. 1981)
American pop star

I always feel I might go either way for a box of chocolate.

LIZ SMITH (B. 1923)
American gossip columnist

The obvious theory behind my fetish is that, since I'm basically afraid of flying, I desire the man who controls the object of fear...an encounter with a pilot is an encounter with an alien, a liaison with a god, an abduction of sorts. The credo among pilots is that you're not truly a member of the mile-high club unless you have sex with the pilot while he's flying the plane.

MEGHAN DAUM (B. 1970)
American writer

Women in the garb of the opposite sex gives rein to the idea that women's sexual fantasy is much broader, and includes a predatory side.

ANNE HOLLANDER (B. 1930)
American writer

Spirits when they please
Can either sex assume,
or both.

JOHN MILTON (1608–1674)
British poet

People ask, "Why do you dress like a woman?"
I don't dress like a woman.
I dress like a drag queen.

RUPAUL (B. 1960)
American performer

A "Bay Area Bisexual" told me I didn't quite coincide with either of her desires.

WOODY ALLEN (B. 1935)
American filmmaker, actor and writer

Like most men, I am consumed with desire whenever a lesbian gets within twenty feet.

TAKI (B. 1937)
Greek-American writer

I have lived and slept in the same bed with English countesses and Prussian farm women…no woman has excited more passions among women than I have.

FLORENCE NIGHTINGALE (1820–1910)
American nursing pioneer

The Butch is the ultimate romantic lesbian figure, androgynous to-die-for, an icon of outsider status and forbidden desire.

SUSIE BRIGHT (B. 1958)
American writer, editor

Some women can be completely gay. I'm not one of them. When I do it, though, I like really trashy porno girls. Like porno 44DD, and they have to be really aggressive. Otherwise, why bother?

COURTNEY LOVE (B. 1964)
American musician, actress

The big money's in gay porn. I don't know if I'd be able to do that, though. No self-respecting homosexual would even want me. They'd see my big, hairy, ugly keister on a wide screen and go, 'We're not that gay.'"

RON JEREMY (B. 1954)
American porn star quoted in Michael Musto's Village Voice *column, "La Dolce Musto."*

Yeah, but flip the guy over and I know there'd be takers.

MICHAEL MUSTO'S REPLY

I don't think I'm gay. I don't think I'm straight. I think I'm just slutty. Where's [my] parade?

MARGARET CHO (B. 1968)
American comedian

There is nothing wrong with going to bed with someone of your own sex…. People should draw the line at goats.

ELTON JOHN (B. 1947)
British musician

As she lay there, dozing next to me, one voice inside my head kept saying, Relax…you are not the first doctor to sleep with one of his patients." But another kept reminding me, "Howard, you are a veterinarian."

DICK WILSON (B. 1916)
American actor, comedian

In homosexual sex you know exactly what the other person is feeling, so you are identifying with the other person completely. In heterosexual sex you have no idea what the other person is feeling.

WILLIAM S. BURROUGHS (1914–1997)
American writer

I CAUSED MY HUSBAND'S

HEART ATTACK.

IN THE MIDDLE OF LOVEMAKING,

I TOOK THE PAPER BAG OFF MY HEAD.

HE DROPPED THE POLAROID AND

KEELED OVER AND SO DID THE HOOKER.

IT WOULD HAVE TAKEN ME

HALF AN HOUR TO UNTIE MYSELF

AND CALL THE PARAMEDICS,

BUT FORTUNATELY THE

GREAT DANE COULD DIAL.

JOAN RIVERS (B. 1933)
American comedian

I am always on top. It's
really unfortunate. I am
begging for the man that
can put me on the bottom.
Or the woman. Anybody
that can take me down.

ANGELINA JOLIE (B. 1975)
American actress

If her nails are long,
she might just be lookin'
for a scratchin' post.

SHAR REDNOUR
American writer, film director

Pleasure does not
exist without pain.
Pain and pleasure are
the same emotion.

MARQUIS DE SADE (1740–1814)
French author

*On the mysterious
disappearance of handcuffs
from restraint kits:*
Clearly our crew are so
professional, they practice
restraint procedures
at home.

A BRITISH AIRWAYS SPOKESWOMAN

**I just had (a penis piercing) done,
but I've received differing opinions about
whether I'm going to have trouble with airport
metal detectors. What's the scoop?**

H.J. OF ST. LOUIS, MISSOURI
In a letter to Playboy

You don't appreciate a
lot of stuff in school
until you get older.
Little things like being
spanked every day by
a middle-aged woman:
Stuff you pay good money
for in later life.

EMO PHILIPS
American comedian

One of my students
had a piercing through
her labia. And she told
me about how when you
ride on a motorcycle,
the little bead on the
ring acts like a vibrator.
Her story turned me on
so I did it. I got two.

KATHY ACKER (1947–1997)
American writer, professor

It's been so long since
I made love, I can't even
remember who gets tied up.

JOAN RIVERS (B. 1933)
American comedian

The walls of my apartment
are so thin that when my
neighbors have sex, I have
an orgasm.

LINDA HERSKOVIC
American comedian

What's embarrassing
about phone sex is that
the neighbors can hear me
having sex but they don't
see anyone enter or leave
the apartment.

SUE KOLINSKY
American comedian

I tried phone sex and
it gave me an ear infection.

RICHARD LEWIS (B. 1947)
American comedian

[Cybersex] really doesn't
mean that much, its just
something that's really fun
to do, that leaves no mess,
no side effects, and its the
best form of contraception
you'll ever find.

16-YEAR-OLD AUSTRALIAN GIRL
Quoted in Growing Up Digital
by Don Tapscott

It was great, but
extremely hard to type
with one hand.

25-YEAR OLD MALE RESPONDENT
to a Men's Health *survey about
online sexual relationships*

I believe that organic
sex, body against body,
skin area against skin area,
is becoming no longer
possible, simply because
if anything is to have any
meaning for us it must
take place in terms
of the values and experi-
ences of the media
landscape....

J. G. BALLARD (B. 1930)
British author

I never miss a chance
to have sex or appear
on television.

GORE VIDAL (B. 1925)
American author

Sex on television
can't hurt you unless
you fall off.

ANONYMOUS

I realize my life is unique and some people think it's a publicity stunt. Well, it isn't. The relationship with Sandy, Mandy, Jessica and Brande was a normal one—except it involved five people. They were my girlfriends and I was sleeping with all of them.

HUGH HEFNER (B. 1926)
American magazine publisher

The mind of the person who's interested in legs and feet is very different from the person who's interested in breasts. Breast men tend to be aggressive, outgoing, athletic—whereas people who like the lower body tend to be frightened, introverted. It all has to do with being down on the floor when you're a scared little child and looking up at that big tower of mommy. What's down there—the feet and the legs, that's where the security is.

DIAN HANSON
American erotic magazine editor

There is no unhappier creature on earth than a fetishist who yearns for a woman's shoe and has to embrace the whole woman.

KARL KRAUS (1874–1936)
Austrian journalist

Sex between a man and a woman can be wonder-ful—provided you get between the right man and the right woman.

WOODY ALLEN (B. 1935)
American actor, writer and filmmaker

Si Non Oscillas Noli Tintinnare. (If you don't swing, don't ring).

BRASS PLAQUE ON THE DOOR OF THE PLAYBOY MANSION

The biggest problem with a ménagè a trois is that when it's all over and you open your eyes, they're still there. And you have to say something nice. And you have to wonder if you're a pervert.

LISA CARVER (B. 1969)
American writer

Do Siamese twins count as one or two?

HOWARD STERN (B. 1954)
American radio personality

Certainly nothing is unnatural that is not physically impossible.

RICHARD BRINSLEY SHERIDAN (1751–1816)
British playwright and politician

Of all the sexual aberrations, perhaps the most peculiar is chastity.

REMY DE GOURMONT (1858–1915)
French novelist and critic

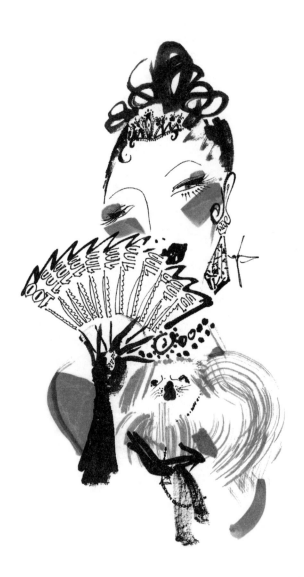

SEX SELLS

The two great obsessions of the modern

world share a fairly large intersection.

Wealth can attract lovers, and wannabe

lovers seek wealth to become more attractive.

Sex can help you sell just about any product,

while some just sell sex itself. Whether they go

hand-in-hand or are making money hand-over-fist

together, the lust for sex and the lust for wealth

make a dynamic couple—and an interesting

topic of discussion.

Money, it turned out, was exactly like sex, you thought of nothing else if you didn't have it and thought of other things if you did.

JAMES BALDWIN (1924–1987)
American writer

My biggest sex fantasy is we're making love and I realize I'm out of debt.

BETH LAPIDES
American comedian

A man wrote me about his girlfriend. Whenever they had sex, she liked to talk finance. She'd say things like, "Come on, baby, let's see you balance my checkbook," or "Oh, honey. Take a loan out for my apartment and pay no interest for six months." Once she shouted, "Mortgage my house payment now!"

DEB LEVINE (AKA ASK DELILAH)
American advice columnist

I'm overdrawn at the bank. I won't say how much, but if you saw it written down, you'd think it was a sex chatline number.

JULIE BURCHILL (B. 1960)
British writer

In sex as in banking there is a penalty for early withdrawal.

CYNTHIA NELMS
American writer

Business is like sex. When it's good, it's very, very good; when it's not so good, it's still good.

GEORGE KATONA (B. 1901)
American economics and psychology professor

Law practice is the exact opposite of sex: even when it's good, it's bad.

MORTIMER ZUCKERMAN (B. 1937)
American businessman

Women prefer men who have something tender about them— especially the legal kind.

KAY INGRAM

All heiresses are beautiful.

JOHN DRYDEN (1631–1700)
English writer

A fool and her money are soon courted.

HELEN ROWLAND (1875–1950)
American journalist

A woman may owe a man a lovin', but not a livin'.

MAE WEST (1893–1980)
American actress, comedian

Beware of the man who praises women's liberation; he is about to quit his job.

ERICA JONG (B. 1942)
American writer

I HATE MY JOB
If you marry me, I can quit. Over-educated, left-leaning, politically-active SWF, 40, seeks SWM. Likes dining out. No one's ever asked me to put a bag over my head. How about you?

FROM *PLAIN FAT CHICK SEEKS GUY WHO LIKES BROCCOLI: 200 PERSONAL ADS*, COLLECTED BY KATHY HINCKLEY

A career is erotically sexual, it's my real passion. A career is like always having a mistress on the side.

RAQUEL WELCH (B. 1940)
American actress

You'd be surprised how much better a man gets when you know he's worth a hundred-and-fifty million dollars.

JOAN RIVERS (B. 1933)
American comedian

For the first time in
Manhattan history,
many women...
have as much money
and power as men—
or at least enough
to feel like they
don't need a man,
except for sex.

CANDACE BUSHNELL
American writer

Losing my virginity was a career move.

MADONNA (B.1957)
American pop star

A lot of girls go out with me just to further their careers. Damn anthropologists.

EMO PHILLIPS
American comedian

She's the kind of girl who climbed the ladder of success wrong by wrong.

MAE WEST (1893–1980)
American actress, comedian

Marie was boss of the whole Personal Injury Department.... She was bossy with Tom, too; she bossed him down one floor into the moldering storeroom for cabinets of dead records whenever she felt the urge [for sex]; she bossed him right upstairs when she was through.

JOSEPH HELLER (1923–1999)
American writer

In the modern workplace, men are drones and women are queen bees.

CAMILLE PAGLIA (B. 1947)
American author, critic and educator

If women can sleep their way to the top, how come they aren't there?

ELLEN GOODMAN (B. 1941)
American newspaper columnist

As for not sleeping with the boss, why discriminate against him?

HELEN GURLEY BROWN (B. 1922)
American editor

The more potent a man becomes in the bedroom, the more potent he is in business.

DR. DAVID REUBEN
American physician and writer

When the stocks go up, the cocks go up!

XAVIERA HOLLANDER (B. 1943)
Dutch prostitute, writer

You don't need a Harvard
M.B.A. to know that the
bedroom and the board-
room are just two sides of
the same ballgame.

STEPHEN FRY (B. 1957)
British actor and writer

Sex! What is that but
[life], after all? We're all
of us selling sex, because
we're all selling life.

ALVIN CHERESKIN
American advertising executive

Corporately, we believe
in orgasms.

WARREN LITTLEFIELD (B. 1952)
American television executive

Money does not corrupt
people. What corrupts
people is lack of affection....
Money is simply the
bandage which
wounded people put
over their wounds.

MARGARET HALSEY (1910–1997)
American writer

**Society drives people crazy with lust and
calls it advertising.**

JOHN LAHR (B. 1941)
American writer, critic

I live for meetings with men
in suits. I love them because
I know they had a really
boring week and I walk in
there with my orange velvet
leggings and drop popcorn
in my cleavage and then fish
it out and eat it. I like that. I
know I'm entertaining them,
and I know that they know.

MADONNA (B. 1958)
American pop star

If widgets sold as well
as sex, I would sell
widgets. But nothing
seems to sell as fast as sex.

SETH WARSHAVSKY (B. 1973)
Internet porn tycoon

Sex is one of the most
wholesome, beautiful
and natural experiences
that money can buy.

STEVE MARTIN (B. 1945)
American comedian, actor

...That delicious,
thrilling, health-restoring
sensation
called vibration...
It makes you fairly
tingle with the
joy of living...

EXCERPTS FROM EARLY 1900'S
AD COPY FOR VIBRATORS
Quoted in The Good Vibrations Guide to Sex

Where there is an ongoing relationship of caring. Where there is a sense of humor. Where there is a sense of mutual mercy. Where there is a sense that God has given sex to you...there is nothing livelier. But when it is merchandised as a commodity for instant gratification, there is nothing deadlier than sex.

WILLIAM SWING (B. 1936)
Episcopalian Bishop of California

When you are in love with someone you want to be near him all the time, except when you are out buying things and charging them to him.

MISS PIGGY
(ACCORDING TO HENRY BEARD)
From the book, Miss Piggy's Guide to Life

Shopping is better than sex. If you're not satisfied after shopping, you can make an exchange for something you really like.

ADRIENNE GUSOFF (B. 1953)
American writer

Advertising didn't mix sex up with our daily lives. The Great Marketeer in the sky did that.

BARRY BROOKS
British advertising executive

If sex did not exist, then a marketing executive would have had to invent it.

GIG MURDOCH (B. 1948)
American businessman, writer

Spanking chic dominates the marketplace these days. Barnes and Noble stocks up for Valentine's Day with Patricia Payne's *Sex Tips from a Dominatrix*. Inept partners bungle with hairbrushes on Ally McBeal. Vodka peddlers shackle their bottles for that Absolut Sadist look. At S&M supper clubs, it's duck for dinner and discipline for dessert. Spanking is hip, and— as with 1970's porno chic, where "nice" couples flocked to see *Deep Throat*— middle-class American consumers are eating it up.

CHRIS DALEY
American writer

Being accused of making money by selling sex in Hollywood, home of the casting couch and the gratuitous nude scene, is so rich with irony that it's a better subject for a comic novel than a column...they're charging Heidi Fleiss with pandering in a town in which the verb is an art form.

ANNA QUINDLEN (B. 1952)
American journalist, author

Leaders of countries called me and asked for sex. You look at any picture of a politician with some girls around him and at least three of them will be mine.... If I really came out and talked, I could have stopped NAFTA.

HEIDI FLEISS (B. 1965)
American entrepreneur known as "The Hollywood Madame")

Our culture uses sex in the most cynical way to "sell" anything— even though we blanch when sex is presented simply, or sold for itself.

SUSIE BRIGHT (B. 1958)
American writer, editor

SEX SELLS

The big difference
between sex for money
and sex for free
is that sex for money
usually costs
a lot less.

BRENDAN BEHAN (1923–1964)
Irish playwright, poet

When I was a call girl, men were not paying for sex. They were paying for something else. They were either paying to act out a fantasy or they were paying for companionship or they were paying to be seen with a well-dressed young woman. Or they were paying for someone to listen to them…. What I did was no different from

Impersonating his mother: Six children, and none of them are married! I've taken the money we've saved on the weddings and I'm using it to build my daughters a whorehouse.

DAVID SEDARIS (B. 1957)
American writer, radio commentator

I enter a whorehouse with the same interest as I do the British Museum or the Metropolitan—

A woman who takes things from a man is called "a girlfriend." A man who takes things from a woman is called "a gigolo."

RUTHIE STEIN
American writer

---

what ninety-nine percent of American women are taught to do. I took the money from under the lamp instead of in Arpege.

ROBERTA VICTOR
American prostitute

Pleasure that isn't paid for is as insipid as everything else that's free.

ANITA LOOS (1893–1981)
American writer

in the same spirit of curiosity. Here are the works of man, here is the art of man, here is his eternal pursuit of gold and pleasure. I couldn't be more sincere.

ERROL FLYNN (1909–1959)
American actor

Oh girls! Set your affections on cats, poodles, parrots or lap dogs; but let matrimony alone. It's the hardest way on earth of getting a living.

FANNY FERN (1811–1872)
America's first advice columnist

DeNiro. While just three years ago Richard Gere bought Julia Roberts for… what was it?… $3,000? I'd say that was real progress.

MICHELLE PFEIFFER (B. 1957)
American actress

If women didn't exist, all the money in the world would have no meaning.

ARISTOTLE ONASSIS (1906–1975)
Greek shipping tycoon

Love is an ocean of emotions entirely surrounded by expenses.

LORD DEWAR (1864–1930)
British industrialist

Love is a costly flower, but one must have the desire to pluck it from the edge of a precipice.

STENDHAL (1783–1842)
French writer

Sex is the great amateur sport. The professional, male or female, is frowned upon; he or she misses the whole point and spoils the show.

DAVID CORT (1904–1983)
American writer

Fifty percent of America's population spends less than ten dollars a month on romance. You know what we call these people? Men!

JAY LENO (B. 1950)
American television host

So this is the Year of the Woman? Well, yes, this has been a very good year for women. Demi Moore was sold to Robert Redford for $1 million. Uma Thurman went for $40,000 to Mr.

Sex—the poor man's polo.

CLIFFORD ODETS (1906–1963)
American playwright, screenwriter

IT'S TRUE THAT THE FRENCH
HAVE A CERTAIN
OBSESSION WITH SEX,
BUT IT'S A PARTICULARLY ADULT
OBSESSION. FRANCE IS THE
THRIFTIEST OF ALL NATIONS;
TO A FRENCHMAN SEX
PROVIDES THE MOST
ECONOMICAL WAY
TO HAVE FUN.

ANITA LOOS (1888–1981)
American novelist, screenwriter

It's amazing how much time and money can be saved in the world of dating by close attention to detail. A white sock here, a pair of red braces there, a grey slip-on shoe, a swastika, are as often as not all one needs to tell you there's no point in writing down phone numbers and forking out for expensive lunches because it's never going to be a runner.

HELEN FIELDING (B. 1959)
British writer

Las Vegas is Everyman's cut-rate Babylon. Not far away there is, or was, a roadside lunch counter and over it a sign proclaiming in three words that a Roman emperor's orgy is now a democratic institution… "Topless Pizza Lunch."

ALISTAIR COOKE (B. 1908)
British writer, historian

If it weren't for pickpockets, I'd have no sex life at all.

RODNEY DANGERFIELD (B. 1922)
American comedian

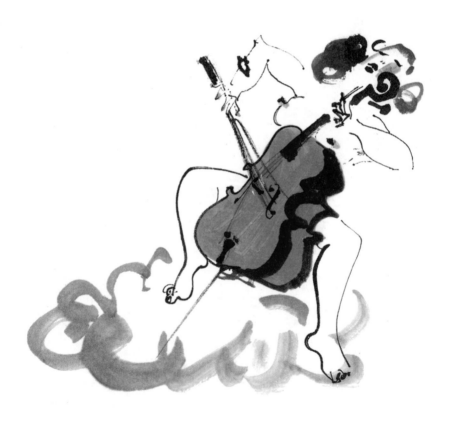

SPIRITUALITY

These days, as many people claim to see
God in their bedrooms as in churches singing
hymns or in their dens listening to old King Crimson
records. Judging by what philsophers, holy men,
and wholly sensual people have had to say on the
subject, maybe it's always been that way.

> **Sex lies at the root of life,**
> **and we can never learn to reverence life**
> **until we know how to understand sex.**
>
> HAVELOCK ELLIS (1859–1939)
> *British physician, writer*

Sex is one of the nine reasons for reincarnation. The other eight are unimportant.

HENRY MILLER (1891–1980)
American novelist

Only death goes deeper than sex.

MASON COOLEY (B. 1927)
American aphorist

Sexual intercourse is kicking death in the ass while singing.

CHARLES BUKOWSKI (1920–1994)
German-born American writer and poet

When people shout, "Oh, God! Oh, God! I'm comin!!" while approaching orgasm, they are not bluffing. Sexual climax is as close as we get to God before our ultimate climax: death.

PHIL MARQUIST (B. 1963)
American writer

Death is orgasm is rebirth is death is orgasm.

WILLIAM S. BURROUGHS (1914–1997)
American writer

On the brink of being satiated, desire still appears to be infinite.

JEAN ROSTAND (1894–1977)
French biologist

Sex has become the religion of the most civilized portions of the earth. The orgasm has replaced the Cross as the focus of longing and the image of fulfillment.

MALCOLM MUGGERIDGE (1903–1990)
British writer

I was wondering today what the religion of the country is, and all I could come up with was sex.

CLAIRE BOOTHE LUCE (1903–1987)
American playwright and ambassador

Sex is not some sort of pristine, reverent ritual. You want reverence and pristine, go to church.

CYNTHIA HEIMEL
American writer, humorist

Your orifice, my oracle.

HARRY HOWITH (B. 1934)
Canadian poet

I like my pussy. Sometimes I stare at in the mirror while I'm undressing. I love my pussy. It's the complete summation of my life…. My pussy is the temple of learning.

MADONNA (B. 1958)
American pop star

To have anonymous sex in a dark alleyway is to pay homage to the dream of male freedom. The unknown stranger is a wandering pagan god. The altar, as in prehistory, is anywhere you kneel.

CAMILLE PAGLIA (B. 1947)
American author, critic and educator

There are things that happen in the dark between two people that make everything that happens in the light seem all right.

ERICA JONG (B. 1942)
American writer

To love deeply in one direction makes us more loving in all others.

MADAME SWETCHINE (1782–1857)
French writer

The grasp divine, th' emphatic, thrilling squeeze
The throbbing, panting breasts
and trembling knees,
The tickling motion, the enlivening flow,
The rapturous shiver and dissolving—Oh!

JOHN WILKES (1725–1797)
English political leader

THE GOOD IS ONE THING;
THE SENSUOUSLY PLEASANT
ANOTHER. THESE TWO,
DIFFERING IN THEIR ENDS, BOTH
PROMPT TO ACTION.
BLESSED ARE THEY THAT
CHOOSE THE GOOD;
THEY THAT CHOOSE THE
SENSUOUSLY PLEASANT
MISS THE GOAL.

FROM THE KATHA UPANISHAD

Sensuality reconciles us with the human race. The misanthropy of the old is due in large part to the fading of the magic glow of desire.

ERIC HOFFER (1902–1983)
American writer

To hear many religious people talk, one would think God created the torso, head, legs and arms, but the Devil slapped on the genitals.

DON SCHRADER
American model, writer

Sex pleasure in woman…is a kind of magic spell; it demands complete abandon; if words or movements oppose the magic of caresses, the spell is broken.

SIMONE DE BEAUVOIR (1908–1986)
French novelist and essayist

At the end of the sexual seeker's journey, there sometimes seems to be an erotic whoopee cushion. How many times have we shaken our heads at our folly? How often does a

Sex is God's joke on human beings.
BETTE DAVIS (1908–1989)
American actress

I would say that the sexual organs express the human soul more than any other limb of the body. They are not diplomats. They tell the truth ruthlessly.

ISAAC BASHEVIS SINGER (1904–1991)
American writer

A standing prick has no conscience.

ENGLISH PROVERB

sexual high come down like a bad acid hangover? I thought I saw God, but it was really a pimple on my ass.

SUSIE BRIGHT (B.1958)
American writer, editor

If a man has a right to find God in his own way, he has a right to go to the Devil in his own way also.

HUGH HEFNER (B. 1926)
American magazine publisher

Women give themselves
to God when the devil
wants nothing more
to do with them.

SOPHIE ARNOULD (1740–1802)
French singer

God and I have a great relationship but we both see
other people.

DOLLY PARTON (B. 1946)
American singer/songwriter

A maiden's chastity is
a sty in the devil's eye.

IRISH PROVERB

human of vital signs.
For them, sex is a form
of enthusiasm, a personal
playground, a team sport,
a wellspring of intimacy,
chuckles, and ecstasy.

JAMES R. PETERSEN
American writer

I remember lovemaking
as an exploration of sadness
so deep that people must
go in pairs….

JOHN UPDIKE (B. 1932)
American writer

**I don't believe in God, but women and trees
are the proof of His existence.**

JEANLOUP SIEFF (1933–2000)
French photographer

To err is human—but it
feels divine.

MAE WEST (1893–1980)
American actress

There are those who
embrace sex, who play
with the danger, who pass
through the keyhole into
a universe of pleasure.
They swim laps in the
"sea of provocation" and
consider "genital commo-
tion" to be the most

Sex is the last refuge
of the miserable.

QUENTIN CRISP (1908–1999)
British writer

There is but one temple
in the Universe…and
that is the human body.
Nothing is holier than
that high form. We touch
heaven when we lay our
hand on the human body.

THOMAS CARLYLE (1795–1881)
British historian

*Perhaps the best function
of parenthood is to teach
the young creature
to love with safety, so that
it may be able to venture
unafraid when later emotion
comes; the thwarting of the
instinct of love is the root
of all sorrow, and not sex only,
but divinity itself, is insulted
when it is repressed.*

FREYA STARK
British travel writer

> THE SPIRIT IS MOST OFTEN FREE
> WHEN THE BODY IS SATIATED WITH PLEASURE;
> INDEED, SOMETIMES THE STARS SHINE
> MORE BRIGHTLY SEEN FROM THE GUTTER
> THAN FROM THE HILLTOP.
>
> W. SOMERSET MAUGHAM (1874–1965)
> *British writer*

Please get over the notion that your particular "thing" is something that only the deepest, saddest, the most nobly tortured can know. It ain't. It's just one kind of sex—that's all. And, in my opinion, the universe turns regardless.

LORRAINE HANSBERRY (1930–1965)
American dramatist

We are each of us angels with one wing, and we can only fly embracing each other.

LICIANO DE CRESCENZO
Italian writer, director and actor

The sexual embrace can only be compared with music and with prayer.

HAVELOCK ELLIS (1859–1939)
English physician and writer

When my house burned down, a friend sent out an e-mail suggesting people dedicate an orgasm to me. A lot of people did. The erotic prayer provided an amazing cushion. I felt so little pain.

ANNIE SPRINKLE (B. 1954)
American porn star

Spiritual beings are also sexual. It's an aspect of being human. I believe posing for Playboy was definitely part of my life's path—I was meant to do it, maybe to set an example for other people, to help other people. It was my fate.

TISHARA COUSINO (B. 1978)
Model

Yoga is a very sexy way
to work out. I think
that anyone who pretends
yoga's not about sex
is just lying to you,
and if they're saying,
"It's very spiritual," well,
it's not as if spirituality
and sex aren't connected.

BETH LAPIDES
American comedian

Sexuality isn't worth a hair
more than spirituality, and
it's the same the other way
around. It's all one, everything is equally good.

HERMANN HESSE (1877–1962)
German-Swiss writer

Tell me who you love, and
I'll tell you who you are.

CREOLE PROVERB

Religion is probably,
after sex, the second
oldest resource which
human beings have
available to them for
blowing their minds.

SUSAN SONTAG (B. 1933)
American writer

All religions have problems
with sex. Sex is at the heart
of people's identity and God
is the symbol for ultimate
meaning. These things are
always intertwined.

JOHN SPONG (B. 1931)
American Episcopalian bishop

Of the delights of this
world, man cares most for
sexual intercourse. Yet he
has left it out of his heaven.

MARK TWAIN (1835–1910)
American writer, humorist

The intimacy in sex is never only physical.
In a sexual relationship we may discover who
we are in ways otherwise unavailable to us,
and at the same time we allow our partner
to see and know that individual. As we unveil
our bodies, we also disclose our persons.

DR. THOMAS MOORE
American theologian, writer

Catholic guilt is definitely a weird aphrodisiac. Once you start getting turned on, you know being bad, and now you're outside the law and outside the blessings of God. You're in the devil's camp, and you might as well just go all the way. Sex for a lot of us is like being thrown off a cliff.

LISA CARVER (B. 1969)
American writer

Who would have ever thought you could die from sex? It was much more fun when you only went to hell.

JOHN WATERS (B. 1946)
American filmmaker

Good girls go to heaven, bad girls go everywhere.

HELEN GURLEY BROWN (B. 1922)
American editor

There is only one real antidote to the anguish engendered in humanity by its awareness of inevitable death: erotic joy.

BENEDIKT TASCHEN
German publisher

If a thing loves, it is infinite.

WILLIAM BLAKE (1757–1827)
English poet

Sex will outlive us all.

SAMUEL GOLDWYN (1879–1974)
American movie mogul

...a more perfect delight
when we be naked in each other's
arms clasped together toying
with each other's limbs, buried
in each other's bodies, struggling,
panting, dying for a moment.
Shall we not feel then, even then,
that there is more in store for us,
that those thrilling writhings
are but dim shadows of a union
which shall be perfect?

SUSAN CHITTY
English writer

INDEX

143